AF000348

PRAGMATIC
KARATE

Traditional techniques and
their value in everyday life

MARK JENNINGS

PRAGMATIC KARATE

Traditional techniques and
their value in everyday life

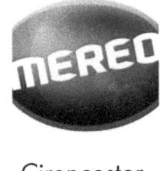

Cirencester

Published by Mereo

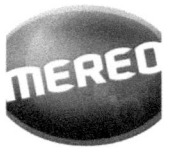

Mereo is an imprint of Memoirs Publishing

25 Market Place, Cirencester, Gloucestershire GL7 2NX
Tel: 01285 640485, Email: info@mereobooks.com
www.memoirspublishing.com, www.mereobooks.com

Copyright ©Mark Jennings, April 2013

The moral right of Mark Jennings to be identified as the author of this work has been asserted by him in accordance with the Copyright, Designs and Patents Act, 1988

First published in England, April 2013

Book jacket design Ray Lipscombe

ISBN 978-1-909544-57-4

All rights reserved.

No part of this publication may be reproduced, stored in a retrieval system, or transmitted in any form or by any means, electronic, mechanical, photocopying, recording or otherwise without the prior permission of Memoirs.

Although the author and publisher have made every effort to ensure that the information in this book was correct when going to press, we do not assume and hereby disclaim any liability to any party for any loss, damage, or disruption caused by errors or omissions, whether such errors or omissions result from negligence, accident, or any other cause. The views expressed in this book are purely the author's.

Printed in England

Disclaimer

Pragmatic Karate is intended as a reference text for those already involved in the practice of martial arts. All practice of martial arts and fighting techniques should always be undertaken under the direct supervision of a qualified instructor.

Neither the author nor the publishers accept any liability or responsibility for any loss or injury arising from the practice of any of the techniques or suggestions mentioned herein.

Contents

FOREWORD - A personal journey
INTRODUCTION - Karate-Do

Part 1 - THE EXTERNAL
Chapter 1:	Mobility	Page 1
Chapter 2:	Striking techniques	Page 9
Chapter 3:	Anatomy and strategy	Page 34
Chapter 4:	Going to the ground	Page 52
Chapter 5:	A modern Interpretation of Karate ni sente nashi	Page 59

Part 2 - THE INTERNAL (mindful self-protection)
Chapter 6:	Zanshin and Mushin	Page 65
Chapter 7:	The ego	Page 70
Chapter 8:	"Positive" and "negative" ego	Page 74
Chapter 9:	Controlling the ego	Page 78
Chapter 10:	Fear	Page 85
Chapter 11:	Future "Fears"	Page 91
Chapter 12:	Now is all there is	Page 96
Chapter 13:	The perils of preoccupation	Page 103

Part 3 - EXTERNAL TECHNIQUES FOR DEVELOPING THE INTERNAL
Chapter 14:	The list	Page 111
Chapter 15:	The commentary	Page 115
Chapter 16:	Routine	Page 120
Chapter 17:	Making yourself a harder target	Page 124
Chapter 18:	Identifying areas of heightened risk	Page 133
Chapter 19:	At home	Page 138

Conclusion: Part 1
A brief, pragmatic look at the twenty guiding principles   Page 143

Conclusion: Part 2
Your Karate-do   Page 154

Glossary   Page 159

Bibliography and suggested further reading   Page 171

FOREWORD

A personal journey

Before we move onto the karate, it may be appropriate to tell you a little about myself, as my views on karate have been influenced by my life away from the dojo as much as they have by my training within it.

My martial arts training began at the age of eight, in the late seventies. Unlike many who began training around that time, I had never seen a Bruce Lee film (although, strangely, I had some of his posters on my wall) and was not really influenced by any celluloid exploits. Videos had yet to be invented and all films were either X or AA certificate and had not been released long enough for one the three channels on TV to have snapped them up.

My training began because, when I was a child, I managed to make enemies of some children who were older and more capable than I which, not surprisingly, led to one or two of them wanting to do me some harm. It was after one such incident that my father decided I needed to learn to defend myself and I was promptly despatched to the local judo club. I practised the judo for a while, but for whatever reason, it never really clicked with me. The instructor was excellent and the other students were friendly, but there was something telling me that it was not for me. I must have been too young to appreciate what it had to offer, as I love watching Judo bouts now.

Around this time, a poster appeared in a local shop for a karate club starting two evenings a week at the local primary school where I was a pupil. After badgering my parents, I eventually attended my first karate class without knowing exactly what karate was. This was the nucleus of what was to become a (so far) lifelong obsession.

Through the eighties I worked my way up through the belts and eventually gained my shodan in 1985 two months after my sixteenth birthday. In those days I was a skinny, long-limbed individual and fell victim to the allure of spectacular, but not always practical, kicking techniques.

In those days, sparring sessions were a little on the excessive side. Minimal padding was worn and the level of contact basically depended on an unspoken agreement between you and your opponent, which was established when one of you made first contact. If they went in hard, so did you, and vice versa. As many of my age group or older reading this will recall, this led to black eyes, split lips, bruised ribs and broken knuckles, but we all stupidly took this in our stride and saw it as a minor hazard of pursuing the art. If nothing else, it developed my pain threshold.

Everything about training, apart from five minutes of mokuso at the end of the session, was about the physical, and, to be honest, I still had quite a journey to go on the inside, but that harsh lesson was waiting for me in the future.

I got my first serious wake-up call regarding my technique when I joined the police at nineteen. I quickly realised that the huge, pretty techniques I had spent years perfecting in the dojo were not that good on a dark, wet street in the midst of a group of violent drunks. My colleagues, the ones who had many years of experience more than me, were not traditional martial artists, but they had perfected one or two techniques over the years which always seemed to work all the time.

Obviously, when word gets around about what you do in your spare time, certain things are expected of you. Thankfully, despite my heart hammering and the most severe adrenalin dump I had ever experienced turning my legs to jelly, I managed to emerge from my first scrape unscathed. It was sobering, however, to realise that I had survived it without resorting to any of the techniques from the dojo. We were trained in taiho-jutsu in the police at that time, which was much more grappling-based.

I began to develop two styles of fighting. One was the pretty, sterile, fighting in the dojo, while the other was the much messier, less attractive, ruck and maul as I tried to manhandle and restrain a prisoner. It never occurred to me at the time - it is only with hindsight that I can see this difference.

Looking back, I can also see a difference between my ippon kumite, with its prearranged attacks, and kumite itself. In the former, my techniques involved mostly close range, upper body strikes and, more often than not, I liked to leave my opponent on the floor. Then, barely two minutes after completing these far more street-effective techniques, we were thrown into full kumite and I would be throwing my legs all over the place again.

Fate was soon to play its hand, however, on two fronts. As far as physical techniques are concerned, the first front, when it came, was an excruciating pain in my upper thigh whilst pad training at a friend's house. It was crippling and the pain remained as a constant companion for some months, and then an occasional visitor for some years. I saw specialists, both Western and Eastern, but nothing seemed to cure it. I eventually found out that it was sciatica, plain and simple. The problem was not my leg at all, it was my lower back.

Knowing this meant that I could gradually tweak my training until everything that aggravated my sciatica would be removed. One aspect which needed to go early on was throwing kicks into fresh air. So, in one fell swoop, one of my main weapons during kumite in the dojo was taken from me and my training, and my views on it gradually began to change.

The second front concerned my internal experience and was the single most traumatic experience of my life, and also one of the experiences which has had the most long-term profound effect upon me.

I mentioned earlier in this chapter that I still had a way to go as far as embracing the philosophy of karate-do was concerned. The event that formed the catalyst for the beginning of my internal journey was not pleasant, but relating it is essential if you are to understand how and why I have changed so much over the years.

On 7th February 1994 I was in uniform and on routine mobile patrol with my colleague PC 3360 Gina Corin Rutherford. It was 4.45 in the morning and we were nearing the end of a night shift which had been quiet, and hence had felt interminable. It was bitterly cold.

The car I was driving hit a patch of black ice and the car simply floated out of my control - it was totally unresponsive. It briefly hit bare tarmac again and gained some traction but immediately hit another patch of ice. This one carried us across to the other side of the carriageway, off the road and over a banking into the River Dearne.

I found out later that the car had hit a pile of tyres just beneath the surface of the water, which caused it to roll forwards onto its roof, smashing the front windscreen in the process and flooding the interior of the car.

As the car was rolling I can remember feeling an intense need to get out of the car, and without thinking I unclipped my seatbelt. This had the effect that the car rolled over and I managed to stay upright as it moved around me.

I remember feeling Gina's arms hitting my legs under the water and grabbed one to try and pull her up, but she slipped from my grasp (she had actually not been able to uncouple her seat belt and was trapped by her own bodyweight as she was upside down).

I am quite tall and was trapped within the confines of the car with my legs between the front seats, and my head pushed up against the back seat where the backrest met the seat proper. The water continued to rise. When it reached my chin, I was forced to pull the upright of the back seat away from the base so I could push by my head into the boot above the water.

I have lost a few seconds after this (I actually think I only remember as much as I do because I was told by a therapist to tell the story as often as possible) and I have no recollection of how much time passed, as my mind has seen fit to erase a segment of the incident. I eventually got out of the car by pulling the rear door handle and hitting the door over and over until it opened enough for me to squeeze through.

Tragically, Gina drowned in that accident. For years I carried with me a morbid view of life, always looking on the darker side of things, always expecting the worst and above all, not really living.

I noticed that my thoughts were bleakest first thing on a weekday morning as I got ready for work and drove into town. I would ponder the inevitability of my own death to an unhealthy degree.

The feeling disappeared as soon as I started interacting with other people. At weekends, this feeling never manifested itself, but I would become morose and moody, as though my mind was trying to sabotage my days when I should have been happiest (I spend my weekends with my wife and daughter).

It was only in the last few years, having read countless self-help books (a nod goes out here to Dan Millman's Way of the Peaceful Warrior, an absolute classic that helped me out no end, thank you) researching various faiths and belief systems and having counselling that I realised it was not some deep psychological damage that had been done, it was, quite simply, once you cut through the extraneous symptoms and reached the root of the problem, guilt.

It was guilt that I had survived whilst poor Gina had not. It was guilt that I had been driving. Could I have done anything differently? (Apart from maybe taking a different route back to the police station, the answer is no). I had not been speeding, I had been doing 37.5 miles an hour in a national speed limit zone, so I was actually well under the speed limit. It was a set of factors that came into play that could not be foreseen and could not have been planned for.

I still feel a deep sadness that Gina passed away, and my heart still goes out to her family. She was only twenty-six years old and had only done about eighteen months in the job. Such a sudden and horrific loss.

I gave my daughter the middle name of Corin as a tribute to her and I won't ever forget, but there is a need to accept that sometimes, bad things do happen to good people for no fathomable reason and there is nothing you can do about it. Accepting this harsh reality helped me greatly in my long (and at the time of writing, still ongoing) healing process.

It also led to a deeper, more profound change. Buddhism began to resonate with me in my aforementioned trawl through faiths and, whilst I am not attached to any temple and have not undergone any initiation, I do consider myself to have Buddhist beliefs (it is quite surprising that, for a faith which considers that attachment leads to suffering, in order for you to be recognised as a Buddhist, the first thing many groups stipulate is that you must attach yourself to them). For me, it matters not where you go to adhere to your faith, what matters is what takes place on the inside and I feel this is true for all religions and beliefs.

One aspect of Buddhism calls for honest self analysis and taking the emphasis off the self (as the self as we understand it does not really exist). Honest self analysis is one of the most difficult things you could force yourself to do and, sure enough, when I had a long hard look at my past behaviour, I would inwardly cringe. It must be realised that you are viewing a younger, less experienced version of yourself through older wiser eyes, so you give your younger self a little leeway, but it is still very uncomfortable.

Taking the onus away from the self and attempting to view the world through the eyes of others causes a shift in your psyche. You see yourself as others see you, and this can be a sobering experience.

Ironically, the experience related above, which I consider to be my most profound lesson in karate, had nothing to do with physical techniques. It occurred on a dark, freezing cold morning and by rights, I should have died. This was just about as far removed from a bright, sterile dojo as you can get.

So, what follows, therefore, covers the general physical training of karate, not so much the bunkai of kata, but the actual physical execution of general techniques and the way they are taught, and an analysis of how the discipline of karate and the mental and philosophical sides of the art still have a place in our current society.

Whilst aimed at practitioners of karate, particularly Japanese-based styles, I would like to think that there is also something here for the lay person who possesses a curiosity towards not just karate, but towards general self protection too.

At the very least, this account of my perception of karate may give you food for thought. At the most, it may have an impact on the way you train, take your training beyond physical technique, and into other aspects of your life.

INTRODUCTION

Karate-Do

Karate-do, the way/art of empty hand fighting, spread outwards during the course of a single century from a small island in the Ryukyu archipelago to encompass the world. It is an art applauded and derided in just about equal measure.

Through shrewd marketing and transformation the art was made palatable by the Okinawan *sensei*, most notably Master Itosu and Master Funakoshi, to the population of Japan. The Japanese overcame the general xenophobia in the aftermath of World War II to make it palatable in turn to huge swathes of the population of the Western World.

Occupying Allied forces found diversions from the confines of their duties so far from home by embracing this small slice of eastern culture, which was of obvious interest to fighting men, giving them an outlet for their stress and aggression during a time of peace.

Then, during the sixties, organisations such as the Japan Karate Association developed a crop of élite *sensei* through their gruelling, now legendary, instructor's programme, and sent them out into the world to spread karate.

The rest, as they say, is history. During the sixties, seventies and eighties the art continued to grow and gain favour steadily throughout the West, which began to develop high quality sensei of its own, ensuring continued growth.

But then, an insidious downfall seemed to begin. Westerners were more interested in the marketability of the art than maintaining its origin. In the West we are all about fast results. People jump from one crash diet to the next, hoping for the miracle rapid weight loss without the torture of exercise even though their subconscious correctly informs them each time that the diet offering the fast results will not deliver on its promise and, in some cases, will actually have an adverse effect on their health. The same became true of karate.

Black belts, once so coveted and worked for over so many years of diligent training, were offered in a fraction of the time. There was a time when the wearing of the black belt came with responsibility and due to the years of experience and hard training the wearer had undergone, that responsibility was more often than not fulfilled.

What many students in pursuit of this innocuous-looking length of black cotton failed to realise was that the obtaining of the *shodan* was actually the start of the serious training, not the climax, when all the subtleties that separated master from student could be studied. The problem was that many sensei who bestowed these black belts upon their hard-working students were not really equipped to deliver this next, higher level of training and a plateau was reached where the skills already acquired would be polished to the *nth* degree, but further development would be in short supply.

Please bear in mind that these statements speak of a general trend and that, just as there are rotten apples in every barrel, I am in no way implying that *all* western *sensei* were of this ilk.

Another problem occurred relating to the sporting aspect of the art. My intention is not to denigrate this exciting and valuable aspect of karate, and I have nothing but respect for the competitors. No, the problem lay in the perception of the techniques.

Formerly effective street techniques had to be outlawed for competition and less practical, but far more spectacular, techniques, began to emerge. All good *karateka* knew the distinction between sport karate and traditional karate and were well aware where the line was drawn between what worked in the tournament and what worked on the street. (There was, in those days, a general lack of understanding of the subtleties of *kata* and an accordingly limited view of the possible applications of the techniques.)

The more spectacular techniques, which looked so good in the sporting arena, also translated well to celluloid, and former sporting champions found themselves embraced as movie stars. Thanks to seeing these films, ironically, *dojo* began to fill with children (and adults) who wanted to emulate their screen idols and thought that, because the technique worked outside for their heroes, it would also work for them. Sensei, quite naturally, taught these techniques, as that is what got the paying public through the door.

Some tried to translate their art to the streets and made it effective, while many more suffered the agony (quite literally) of defeat. The ones that were successful discovered that they could tweak the art to fit into the streets, possibly not realising that what they had been taught was already adapted from the original art and their ultimate destination was not too far from where karate originated. The journey they took made them into some of the best instructors that we have in the world today, but their arduous journey might well have been smoother (and less painful) if not for this blurring between the two aspects of the art.

Strangely, styles which were still based around Okinawa, such as Goju-Ryu, continued to train in the art as a form of combat plain and simple and, whilst their growth was not as rapid as the styles which were imported to Japan, their influence now reaches just as far.

Another hard blow came with the advent of the Ultimate Fighting Championship. The lure of different disciplines coming together in combat was just what martial artists the world over had been waiting for. The somewhat narrow-minded argument over which art is best had been discussed and debated for a long time.

(The short answer to this by the way, is that *no* art is better than any other. It is the students who are better or worse and, until they perfect cloning so that the same person can be trained in two different arts for the same length of time and intensity, the above argument is moot).

However futile, the debate raged on. But what the general public failed to account for was that the martial artists, including *karateka*, who entered the tournaments were doing so utilising the *sporting* techniques. Not surprisingly, when they encountered fighters who did not keep their distance but closed in and dragged them to the ground, they found themselves swiftly despatched. This led to a general public opinion (a flawed opinion, in my view) that karate was not effective. Even now, when Lyoto Machida delivers a knee strike, they say he has borrowed it from Muay Thai when, in all honesty, he will see it as a *hiza-geri*.

Both he and Anderson Silva were lauded for the "front kicks" they employed to win fights. These were apparently passed on from the actor Steven Seagal, a man well versed in Japanese martial arts, who did not refine their teep but their *mae geri*.

Now we have 'mixed martial arts', a general term for a hybrid of different systems brought together so the fighter can cross disciplines and move easily from striking to grappling and standing to ground fighting. I greatly enjoy watching MMA and have followed the UFC since its inception. There are some truly great fighters out there, but I wonder how many of them, if they actually studied a traditional art as it was originally taught, would find that they do not need to cross disciplines at all and would actually find everything they need in

one place? After all, wrestling originally contained strikes, and the majority of striking arts originally contained grappling techniques.

The problem with traditional martial arts is that they were originally developed for fighting, not as a sport, but as a life or death struggle. With the advent of a more modern age (I refuse to use the term "more civilised", simply because we are not) the former battlefield arts were preserved by being formalised.

When karate, a civilian self-defence system for use against untrained attackers, came to Japan, it too was transformed from *jutsu* to do. The irony of it is that an argument could be put forth that, without this transition, the art would not have spread as far across the world as it did.

Fortunately, a renaissance has been occurring over the past ten or twenty years whereby the art is being newly explored and the subtleties are being rediscovered. *Bunkai* and *oyo* are now becoming integral forms of training for many *karateka* and their healthy exchanges of ideas across different styles and disciplines have led to renewed interest in their traditional arts.

But what of the philosophy? If you read Master Funakoshi's biography, *Karate-Do My Way of Life* (see bibliography) you will find that he was held in high esteem by his neighbours and was called on for his wise counsel just as much as his prowess as a fighter, if not more. This is due to his pursuit of the art reaching far further than just techniques in the dojo and seeping into the way he lived his life.

This would have been by design, not accident. He saw his art as a way of life, something which transcends mere physical technique. How many of us today who practise the art of karate actually do so as a way of life? I have concerns that, whilst the necessary and much needed renaissance regarding the effectiveness of technique is taking place, the philosophy and more far-reaching aspects of karate may be neglected.

Part 1
THE EXTERNAL

Chapter 1

Mobility

Throughout this text I may regularly refer to the Shotokan style of karate, as that is obviously where the majority of my experience lies, but the principles discussed can also be applied to other styles.

Have you ever noticed that during a traditional karate class, the stances are rigidly adhered to during *kihon* and *kata*, but as soon as the students start practising *kumite*, the stances become more shallow, the grip on the floor is relaxed somewhat and the weight distribution changes? This is simply because standing in a deep, rigid stance effectively renders you immobile and exposed.

Line Training

With the sudden increase in numbers of people practising the art of karate, the old system of one-to-one tuition was no longer feasible and a method had to be devised for many to be trained by few. This led to the birth of line training as we know it. The students would line up facing the *sensei*, with beginners to his/her right proceeding in order to advanced grades to his/her left. The class would then commence with *kihon* and the students would traverse the dojo, practising the given technique until the walls stopped them, and then turn around and go back the other way.

CHAPTER I

Now, whilst moving in stance like this certainly builds a strong and flexible lower body, the fact is that during one-to-one *kihon* training, this would not have been done. The technique would have been executed from *shizentai* and then back again. *We were never meant to move in a straight line from one stance to the next.* This practice gives ammunition to the critics of Shotokan, who perceive it as an immobile style. This has been exacerbated by the pursuit of deeper and deeper stances.

The Hara or Tanden

I have heard both of the above terms used to refer to this part of the body and it is also referred to as *tantien* in the Chinese arts. It is a point on your body about three inches below your navel and is, essentially, your centre of gravity.

Putting it simply, if, whilst moving, you keep your *tanden* directly beneath your upper body, you will maintain your balance. When you move, try to imagine that someone is pulling you along with a chord which emanates from your body at your *tanden,* but keep your shoulders in line with it and do not lean back or forwards. The stances can aid in your balance and assist in keeping you centred, but only if they are not too deep.

Stances

Some time ago, I wrote an article which the editors of *Traditional Karate* magazine were kind enough to publish on the subject of Shotokan basic stances. This was at a time when I was trying to justify why we do what we do and my conclusion was that the stances were basically an ideal, when a number of favourable factors come together. What follows is a similar text, but much revised and updated.

CHAPTER I

Shizentai – The ready stance

The first stance anyone learns when they come into a dojo is the simplest, but actually the most important. The karateka stands with feet shoulder width apart and the feet turned slightly inwards. The weight distribution between the feet is even, the muscles of the legs are charged but not tensed and the knees are slightly flexed.

In any real situation, this is the position you would most likely be in immediately prior to physical confrontation taking place. This is, essentially, the springboard from which you can launch any and all of your techniques.

In *The Twenty Guiding Principles of Karate* by Gichin Funakoshi (published by Kodansha International, 2003), the Master states, as principle number seventeen:

"*Kamae* (ready stance) is for beginners; later one stands in *shizentai* (natural stance)."

Now, the subject of karate is vast and covering it with only twenty principles is quite an undertaking. Yet, as one of those principles, Master Funakoshi chose to include a principle which could be interpreted as meaning that advanced grades must fight from *shizentai*.

Think about it for a second. As soon as you get a whiff of trouble, you can correctly distribute your bodyweight and flex your legs, all hidden by your clothing, and giving no hint to your opponent that you are about to move (either to fight or run away). If we were to practise *kihon* line training with this in mind, after every technique, we should step forward into *shizentai* before stepping forward again into the chosen stance to deliver a technique. This would ensure that the student gets used to setting off from the most natural position they could possibly be standing in. It will get them used to gaining power and momentum over a shorter distance, wean them off spending long periods motionless in an impractical stance and alter their mindset where the consideration of stances is concerned.

CHAPTER ONE

Zenkutsu-dachi – The front stance

Following *shizentai*, the students are told to step forward, executing a *gedan-barai* (see chapter three) and landing in *zenkutsu-dachi*, the front stance. This is their *kamae*, as mentioned by Master Funakoshi.

From *shizentai*, the karateka moves the left foot (as it was always left leg first), inwards towards the right and then pushes forwards and out until the foot is once again at shoulder width but now comes to rest approximately two shoulder widths in front of the right foot. The two shoulder widths rule is a conservative estimate as this stance is often seen being executed far deeper. The weight distribution is approximately seventy/thirty in favour of the front leg, which is bent until only the tips of the toes can be seen. The front foot is turned slightly inwards and the back foot is turned outwards.

In the early days the rear leg was kept straight (I can still I remember the rigidity of the rear leg being tested by one of my sensei none too gently when I was younger!) but recently, it has become the norm for the knee to be slightly bent. The hips are either at ninety degrees to the direction of travel or forty five degrees, depending upon the technique being executed.

The students then proceed to move up and down the dojo in this stance, encouraged to keep it deep and not to raise their bodies as they step forward.

The problem with the way this stance is practised is that it is not varied to meet specific needs. The fact that the weight is pushing forwards and the rear foot pushes into the floor to augment the power of the technique does not rely on the depth of the stance, it relies on the body mechanics that moving in this stance as a lower grade should instil in you. The rotation of the hips, the connection to the floor and travelling from the *hara/tanden* are what give the power to your techniques. If you move forward, concentrating on balance and the technique you intend to deliver, the stance will take care of itself. It will not be as deep, but you will move across the floor quicker, be better able to get your bodyweight behind our technique and therefore be able to increase power.

In addition, over the long term, deep stances with weight disproportionately held over one bent leg can be very damaging for the knee joint, as can pushing the knee outwards when dropping into the deep stance.

Kokutsu-dachi – The back stance

After running through the techniques which can be employed from *zenkutsu-dachi*, the students then move on to practice *kokutsu-dachi.*

The karateka, having returned to *shizentai*, brings the left foot in as before but steps forwards with the left foot, keeping it in line with the right heel. The heels remain in this straight line throughout, with the rear foot turned outwards at ninety degrees, the front foot facing forwards and the weight distribution about sixty/forty in favour of the rear leg. The hips are turned in line with the direction of travel.

This stance was actually developed from a far shallower and more manoeuvrable version known as *neiko-ashi-dachi*, or "cat stance" where the feet are nowhere near as far apart and the front foot rests on the ball.

The first glaring question regarding this stance is: how can you move forward in *kokutsu-dachi* in a combat effective manner when most of your weight is on your back leg?

The simple answer is: You can't. No matter how fast you try to do it, moving forward in this stance requires a body weight shift towards your front foot before you can even think about moving. Add the factor that students tried to get as deep as possible again and the mobility problem becomes even worse.

That is because this stance, and the stance upon which it was based, are meant to be performed moving backwards. They are a retreating step, primarily for pulling away from your opponent and dragging them off-balance and towards you. The turning of the hips to bring them in line with the direction of travel aids this. They also lighten the load on the front leg for a defensive kick if required.

Were you to practice this stance in a *dojo*, the most effective way would be to start at the very front of the dojo and move backwards into the stance, stepping back into *shizentai* after each technique.

Once again, if you concentrate on the intent of the stance, pulling back, rotating away from the opponent and slightly down, and concentrating on maintaining your balance through the *hara/tanden*, rather than the exact weight distribution and placement of your feet, you will find that the stance takes care of itself, although it will probably not be as deep.

Incidentally, the *kokutsu-dachi* at the beginning of *Heian Nidan, Sandan, Yondan* and *Godan* should, in my opinion, be executed by stepping backwards.

Kiba-dachi – The Straddle or Horse-Riding Stance

The only time we used this stance during *kihon* when I was young and going through the grades was to practice *yoko-geri*. It really was an underused stance. Bearing in mind that the *Tekki/Naihanchi kata* are made up exclusively of *Kiba-dachi*, this seems quite an anomaly.

The student would turn sideways on, with their left side facing the front of the dojo and feet (at least momentarily) together before stepping into the stance by pushing the left foot out and coming to rest approximately two shoulder widths (again a conservative estimate) away from the right, with the weight distributed evenly. The feet were turned slightly inwards, the knees were pushed out, the back was straight and the buttocks were pushed under (which,

CHAPTER ONE

when you first encounter this stance, is very uncomfortable and is, in truth, unnecessarily complicated.)

The student, when moving in this stance, would stay sideways on to the front of the dojo and step forwards by crossing their feet and then stepping into the next stance with the same front leg as before.

Firstly, the crossing of the feet in any situation is a no-no. It is just about as unbalanced as you can get whilst keeping both feet on the ground. Secondly, once again, the stances are too deep.

Like *kokutsu-dachi*, this stance was adapted to meet the requirements of line training. *Kiba-dachi* is meant to be performed sideways from *shizentai* and is another means of pulling away from your opponent and breaking his balance.

Once again, concentrate on the *hara/tanden*, a sharp sideways movement and a slight drop in height and the stance will take care of itself. After stepping sideways into *kiba-dachi*, bring the rear leg back up into *shizentai*.

I could go on working my way through all the stances available to the *karateka* but, in all honesty, my text would be variations on a theme, as the same principles can be applied to any stance. Although stances are held in such high regard and the pursuit of the perfect stance can take up much of a *karateka's* time, I believe that they arose from the simple, practical requirement that a fighter needs to be able to move in any direction whilst maintaining balance and the ability to apply power to a technique. I also think that this is the reason for the wide variety of stances too, because if you execute a technique fifty times, but concentrate on balance, movement of body weight and the execution of the technique, there is a good chance your feet will end up in fifty slightly different positions. This is what I meant by the formal stances being an ideal.

In addition, you will probably find, as I did, that when you try moving by thinking about the intent behind the technique and the feel of it, rather than concentrating on the deep formal stance, you will move a lot faster. Although *bunkai* falls way outside the scope of this

CHAPTER ONE

book, practising *kata* with the practicality of your stance in mind can completely alter the way you execute it and change the emphasis on techniques, helping you to see new possibilities when searching for the underlying intention in the reason for their execution.

Deeper stances are not only rendering you immobile, they are also having a detrimental effect on your balance. Weight transference from one foot to the other is far easier when the legs are at a more natural distance. For instance, in a formal *zenkutsu dachi*, the body weight is so far forwards that, should your front foot be taken away by *ashi- barai*, or a *gedan mawashi-geri*, the chances of transferring your weight to the other leg are practically non-existent. Now, obviously, if you are travelling in one direction, the foot coming to rest will bear the majority of the weight. It has to in order to provide power for your technique. What I am advocating is travelling just enough to add the power, without compromising your balance.

The performance of techniques in this manner may not be as aesthetically pleasing, especially during *kata* practice, but even though the stances will be shallower, by observing proper technique and balance you can make yourself more mobile and hence, your training more combat effective.

So, worry less about the aesthetics of the stance, try and concentrate on projecting your body weight in the direction of your technique. When engaging in *kihon* do not pull yourself to a stop by locking yourself into stance, but try and maintain a natural feel to your weight distribution and balance. As long as you concentrate on maintaining balance and projecting the power in the right direction you will find that factors like the placement of your feet and the distribution of your bodyweight will take care of themselves.

Chapter 2

Striking techniques

As you have likely gathered by now, during this text, I am assuming that the reader has at least a rudimentary knowledge of the execution of techniques. The mechanics of all the techniques which come under the umbrella of traditional karate have already been covered in many books over the years. In the following chapter I offer slight changes to tweak your techniques, without losing the essence of the art.

Distance

The formalisation of karate training, whilst maintaining the actual techniques either through *kihon* practice or through *kata*, caused one major setback in rendering them combat effective. *It required you to execute them at the wrong distance.*

In traditional *kumite*, the fighters keep a respectful distance from one another, whether it is *ippon kumite* or full freestyle. In an actual confrontation, however, the opponents are more likely to be around eighteen inches apart (if that). This is much closer than any formal training taking place in many traditional dojo. Unfortunately, there is a good chance that the opponent you will likely be facing is in his comfort zone at this distance, having cut his teeth (so to speak) outside, rather than in a relatively safe, sterile dojo environment. What you need to do is tip the scales back in your favour.

CHAPTER TWO

Now the good news. The techniques you have been learning in the dojo were actually meant to be executed at short distances. The distancing used in a traditional dojo is due to the formalised training and deep stances. These afforded more time to execute the techniques, hence allowing aspects to be added to make the techniques look more aesthetically pleasing. It is a well-known maxim that simpler techniques are easier for the student to retain and more effective in live situations, and the paring down and simplification of techniques seems to be at the crux of analysing what changed when karate was made more formal.

Hikite

This is one of the most underused and misunderstood aspects of karate technique. The *hikite* is the "pulling hand" and is the one that seems to either sit on your hip or across your torso during *kihon*. It seems somewhat superfluous, as though the hand and arm are, for the time being at least, redundant and are held in reserve until required once more.

Over the years I have heard it described as "chambering" for your technique, as though this is the optimum position from which to begin any offensive manoeuvre. It is not. Keeping your hand in this position for that purpose, even for a second, during actual conflict exposes the entire side of your body to attack.

The truth is that *hikite* has its uses and is an essential tool in making karate techniques more street effective. The reason that its actual use is neglected in a typical Shotokan dojo is that grappling is rarely if ever practised as part of the art and it is in the realm of vertical grappling that *hikite* comes into its own.

The following are some examples of how *hikite* can be used. Please bear in mind that the use of stances, as explained in the previous chapter, is also relevant to *hikite* as well as the strikes and, although we are dealing with separate issues in isolation, it is only when the composite parts are brought together as a whole that the true effectiveness of techniques is realised.

The group of techniques mentioned here is not exhaustive and I urge you to tinker and experiment on your own. If you intend to practise these, do so slowly with compliance in the beginning.

Defence against a wrist grab

Taiho jutsu was an art of arrest and restraint utilised by those keeping the peace in feudal Japan and typically involved escorting a passive prisoner with one hand on his elbow and one on his wrist. (See Fig 2:1 below).

This is supposed to place the prisoner in a disadvantageous position. The person escorting him is able to read his intentions while staying in touch with his body (for instance, if he tried to set up for a strike) and has placed himself at a distance where he would clearly see any attack and would be able to frustrate it by ruining his prisoner's balance.

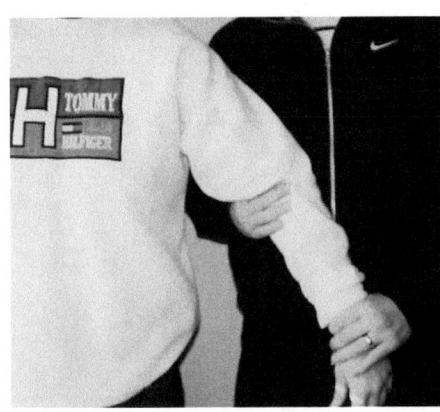

Fig 2:1

If the person being detained shows no signs of aggression, this is the normal carriage position with which they would be escorted. From here, the *taiho jutsu* exponent can escalate accordingly should his detainee become more aggressive by manipulating the elbow and wrist into a variety of restraints, takedowns and strikes to assure compliance through pain and a disadvantageous body position.

Basically, if the person grabbing you is highly skilled in *taiho jutsu* you would be in serious trouble once these two hands are in place.

CHAPTER TWO

If the carriage position were adopted as at Fig 2:1, the best means of escape would be to twist the restrained hand until you could grab their wrist by twisting your hand up and around anti clockwise. Done correctly, this grab can bend the opponents arm into the "S" Lock, which causes a painful rotation of the wrist joint. (The technique of placing an "S" block on your opponents occurs frequently in *kata* - watch out for it.)

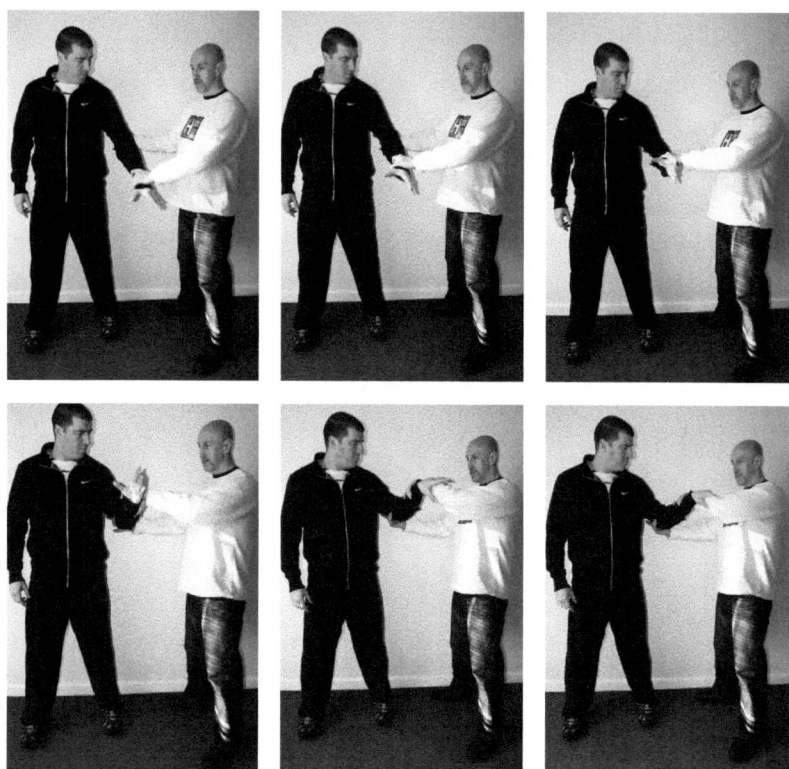

Now, if I lived on a small island that was subjugated by a nation that boasted a warrior caste who favoured these civilian arrest techniques, I would consider a knowledge of escapes from them extremely valuable. Whilst it can be argued that much of karate

CHAPTER TWO

came from Chinese martial arts, there must have been some of the indigenous *Ti* left too. Maybe this is where the *hikite* comes from?

Any right-to-right or left-to-left wrist grab can be dealt with in this manner. It does not have to be under the circumstances of restraint *a la taiho jutsu*.

For a left-to-right wrist grab, the circle executed by your hand to grab the person's wrist is performed the other way and then the opponent is yanked off balance, (see below, Note: in the last image, *uke's* elbow is pushing against that of his opponent to increase the pressure.) The arm position adopted by *uke* is reminiscent of the "hook" strike in the *Tekki/Naihanchi kata*. I urge you to look at other techniques in your *kata* which could be construed as escapes from wrist grabs.)

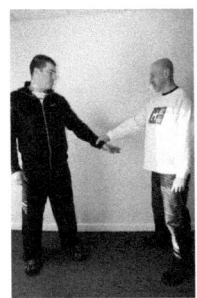 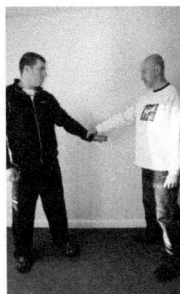 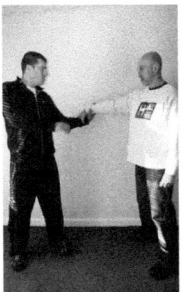 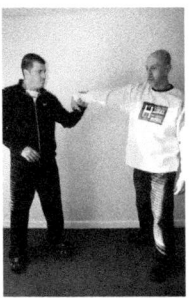

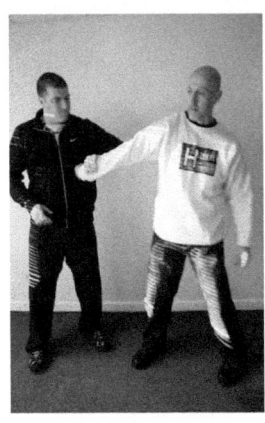 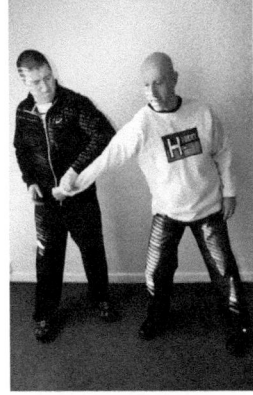 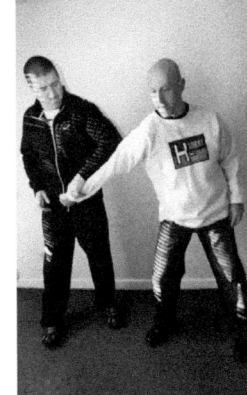

Pulling an opponent off balance by the wrist has to be done fast, heavily and severely. The initial grab has to be quick and the subsequent pull has to follow it immediately.

Defence against a clothing grab

The clothing grab is really a precursor to delivering a strike, whether it is a two-handed grab intended to augment a head butt (Fig 2:2) or a single grab intended to facilitate a punch (Fig 2:3).

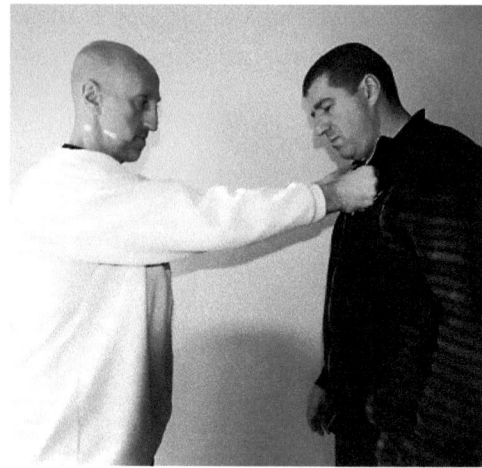
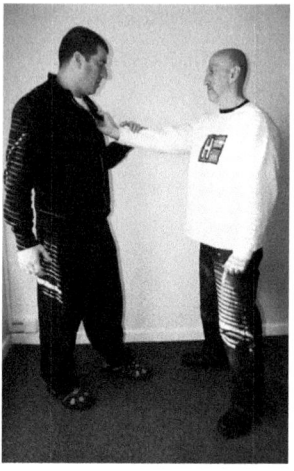

(Fig 2:2)   (Fig 2:3)

CHAPTER TWO

Defending against the two handed grab

For one defence against this grab, the finishing position (prior to the takedown) for the *hikite* resembles the fists on the hip position from numerous *kata* as can be seen in the sequence which follows.

One method for dealing with the two-handed grab would unfold as follows: The opponent has grabbed the *karateka* by the lapels. The *karateka* pulls back and away from his opponent, dropping his vulnerable chin as he does so. He then raises his hands and drops them onto the opponent's forearms. He then reaches over the top with his right hand, delivering a *mawashi empei* on the way across and takes hold of the fleshy part of his opponent's left hand.

By pressing the thumb of his right hand into the back of the opponent's left and pulling the right hand back as he does, coupled with a forceful hip twist, the *karateka* begins to upset the opponent's balance. He then brings his left elbow over the arm of his opponent and pushes down against the elbow joint and the lock is complete.

The beauty of this lock is that it does not matter whether you end up elbow-to-elbow with the opponent or his arm nestles in your armpit, the effect is much the same as long as pressure is exerted on his extended elbow joint.

From here a turn and step to the right brings him to the floor (NB the shrewd observer may notice that this finishing position is reminiscent of the last technique in *Hangetsu;* the wrist of the opponent is bent inwards and the elbow is pushed straight by *uke's* knees so that downwards pressure can be exerted on the shoulder, thereby pinning the opponent's shoulder to the floor. The likeness of these techniques to recurring techniques in traditional *kata* cannot be mere coincidence.)

CHAPTER TWO

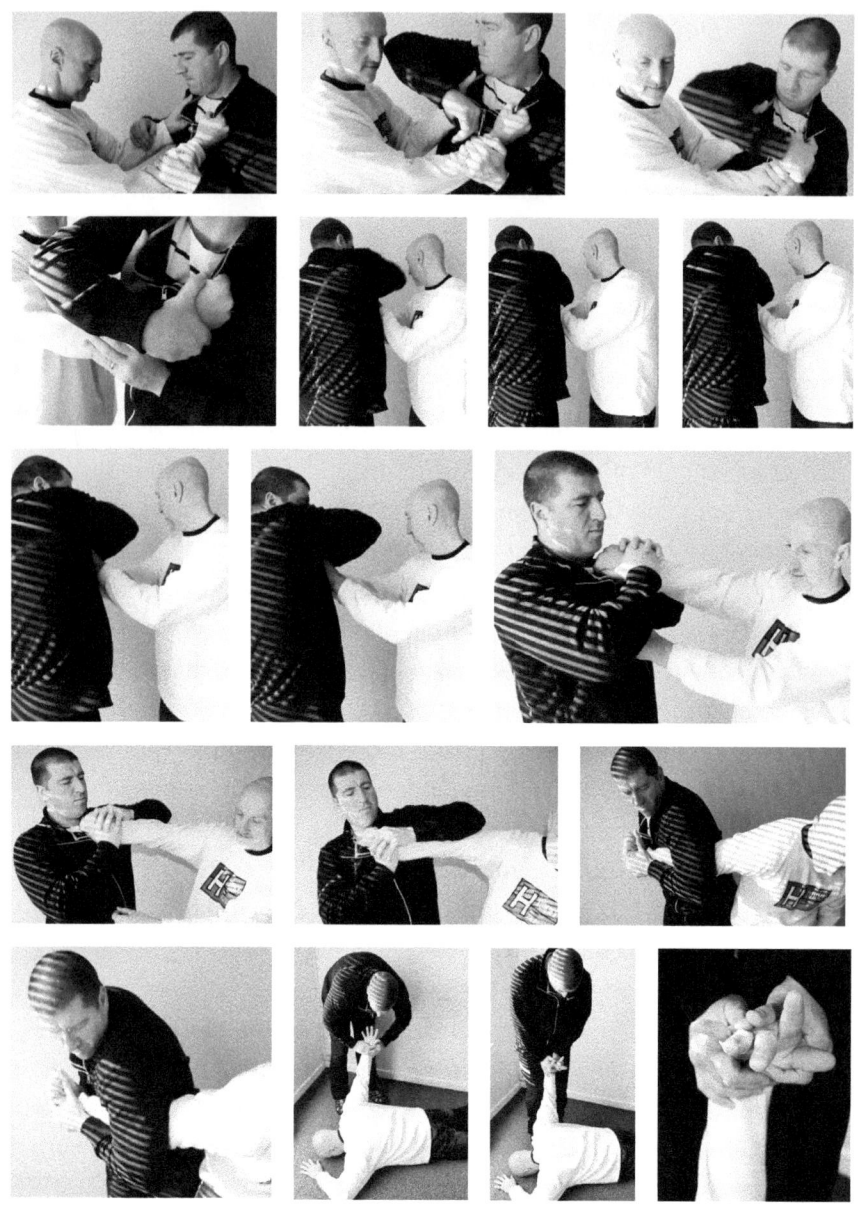

CHAPTER TWO

Defending against the one-handed grab

Although the following technique works just as well with a two-handed grab, I have chosen to show it from the standpoint of being grabbed as preparation for the delivery of a punch, hence one-handed. This technique, it its entirety, is the traditional means of executing *shuto-uke* from beginning to end. It shows the means by which *hikite* can come to rest across the torso.

Once again, our *karateka* is grabbed, this time with one hand. In anticipation of this being a set up for a punch, the *karateka* drops his chin as before and brings his left hand up to the right side of his face (see below). Note: this is not intended as a block, the hand will only be there momentarily. It is just in case. You never know how fast your opponent can be and the hand covering his target area can serve as a distraction.

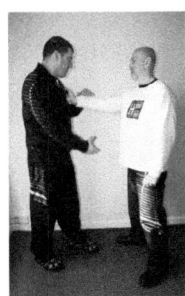
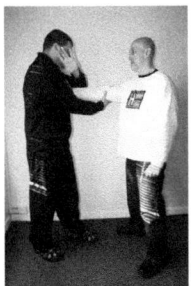
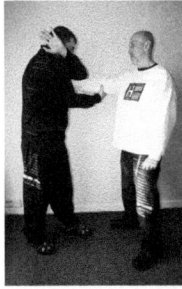
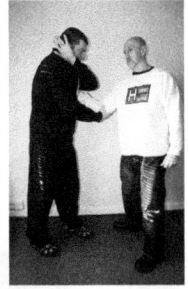
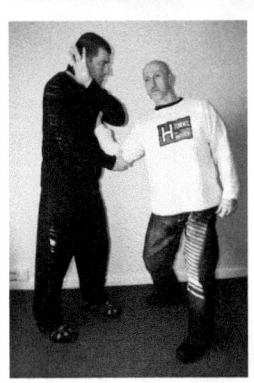
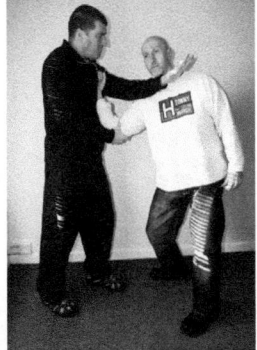
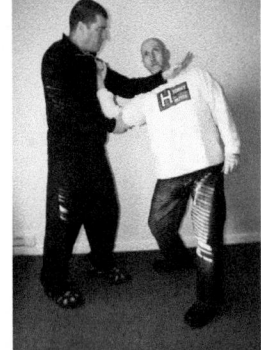

CHAPTER TWO

At the same time as this hand is raised to cover the likely attack site, the *karateka* reaches across with his right hand and takes hold of the opponent's elbow. The karateka then violently wrenches the elbow across to his right at the same time as driving his left hand across to the opponent's face/neck region. This is done to the accompaniment of a backward step and slight body drop as per the previous comments relating to *kokutsu dachi* and *neikoashi dachi*.

The step back and body drop at the same time as the wrench on the elbow greatly upset the opponent's balance and set him up for the strike with the left due to the whiplash on his neck. This is extremely versatile as, depending on the distance, the striking surface used can be anywhere from your elbow downwards (below left) and can even be used in a grappling context (below right).

Hikite can also be used offensively by pulling your opponent onto a technique in order to augment its power. It is the universal law of momentum which is most often demonstrated when vehicles collide. Two vehicles heading towards each other, both travelling at

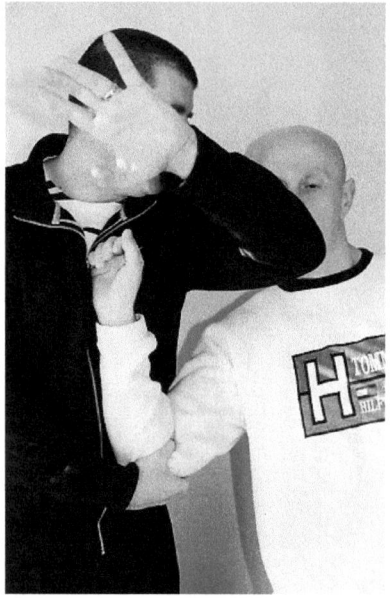 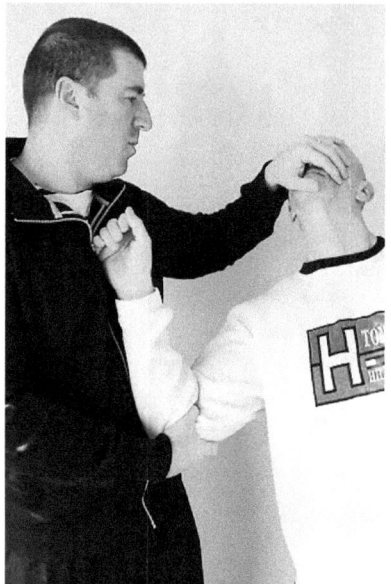

thirty miles per hour will, on impact, have a combined collision velocity of sixty miles an hour. It therefore stands to reason that, should you violently drag your opponent into a technique travelling towards him at speed, its effect will increase exponentially.

Bearing *hikite* in mind, and not merely seeing it as a redundant limb, explore the possibilities for pulling and pushing opponents off balance in preparation to the delivery of your chosen technique.

"Blocks"

Please note the inverted commas. This is because the blocks in traditional karate are more likely misunderstood striking techniques.

As we are working on the theory that our traditional techniques are being executed from the wrong distance, and the actual distance must be much closer, the luxury of time afforded the *karateka* during *ippon kumite* disappears at close range. There is neither the time or the distance to block in most live situations and being solely reliant upon the "block then counter" mindset is, in a real situation, extremely dangerous.

When you look at the basic blocks from a striking perspective, they can be used with or without *hikite* and can have a variety of applications dependant only upon individual preference.

One change that has to occur as far as these techniques are concerned is that their method of execution must be streamlined. The formal techniques carried out in a dojo are too showy and flowery. For instance, let us look at *soto-ude-uke* and *uchi-ude-uke*.

CHAPTER TWO

Soto-ude-uke

Traditionally, when stepping forwards to execute this technique during *kihon*, the blocking arm is pulled all the way back as the *karateka* travels before swinging through a wide arc to intercept the punch at *chudan* level, the mindset being that striking the punching arm with your arm will send it safely off course and render your opponent vulnerable. This is extremely impractical and probably stems from the line-training mentality of travelling in stance. All the pulling back of the arm is merely wasted effort. The same technique can be executed without any extraneous movements - merely raising the arm and twisting the hips would be sufficient and far less time consuming.

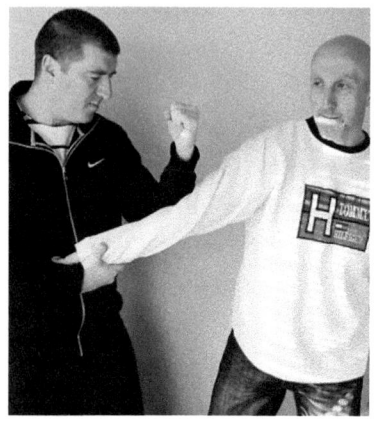

The power and speed of delivery of the technique increases because the striking surface is closer to the body and the twist of the hips is quicker and more pronounced.

Utilising this technique with a strong *hikite* can have a devastating effect on the elbow of an opponent, as long as it is treated as a strike rather than a block.

Uchi-ude-uke

This "block" was always seen by everyone I trained with (and myself) as being such a weak block that it was almost useless. If that was the case, why was it there?

Once again, a technique fell victim to the line training mentality. It was executed by tucking the arm under the opposite arm as the *karateka* stepped forwards before a somewhat ineffectual arc was

CHAPTER TWO

drawn with the fist. The arm position resembled *soto-ude-uke* but was on the opposite side of the torso, the mindset this time being that the outside of the forearm would be used to take the arm away from its target. (The only time this seemed to work, however, was with strong *tai sabaki* which, when doing five step sparring, was not really possible. Thus a mindset that you must remain directly in front of your opponent is deeply embedded even though it is well known that this is flawed.)

The time taken to execute this technique and the ineffectiveness of the actual "block" fairly scream out that it must have had a different original application. The most effective use I have found for this technique is as another defence against a wrist grab.

Now, there can be no aesthetically-pleasing tucking under of the arm. What it needed is for the hand to be whipped upwards in a tight arc. Coupled with a step back and body drop, the power is increased. As the wrist of the opponent is twisted, it causes a bend of the elbow, which causes the shoulder to drop, which exposes his face to a counter. This will either free the *karateka* from the grip or set the opponent up for a strike.

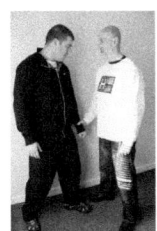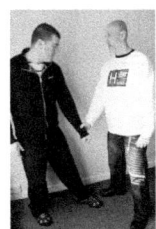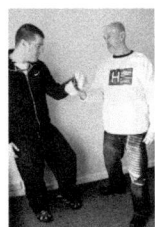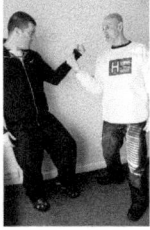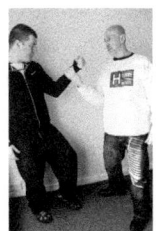

It seems that what "traditional" karate treats as blocks works very well with *hikite* and I would urge you to tinker and experiment in your own time with this.

Please bear in mind that the list is only limited by your own imagination and I am merely imparting a few examples as food for thought.

CHAPTER TWO

Shuto-uke

We have already mentioned that the stance with which this technique is predominantly practised is being executed in the wrong direction. The truth is, it does not have to be executed in *kokutsu dachi*, it can be executed in any stance. In fact, at the risk of upsetting the purists, when moving forwards with this technique during kata, it is best to either shorten your stance back to *neiko ashi dachi* or to forget about stances totally and concentrate on remaining balanced and executing the technique correctly. If you are moving forwards with it in *kata,* there must be a forwards moving application and this does not fit with the "retreating" concept behind *kokutsu dachi.*

One of my favourite *kata* is *Kanku-Dai,* also known as *Kushanku.* This contains a high concentration of *shuto-uke.* If it appears so much in the *kata,* it must a) be seen as very important in actual combat and b) be extremely versatile to appear so many times.

Bearing in mind the use of *hikite* (which does not have to be used every time) and thinking of attacking the arms, neck and head, *shuto* is indeed versatile, but is not a block (see above for examples of its effectiveness, but, as I said, there does not always have to be a *hikite* involved).

Strikes

One aspect of karate which is often commented on is the cultivation of the fist. How to clench it properly, which knuckles to punch with and how to condition them accordingly were all hot topics when I was going through the grades and we used to spend a long time doing press-ups on our knuckles and rubbing them with surgical spirits to toughen the skin.

This adoration of the one strike would lead to a *kamae* stance in freestyle with the fists clenched and the favoured technique in

CHAPTER TWO

tournaments being *gyaku-zuki* (although, again, this had a lot to do with the distancing).

If you immediately clench your fists in a live situation, you place yourself at a disadvantage. Don't get me wrong, punches are a highly effective weapon when used correctly and I am not for one minute suggesting that they should not be used. What I am suggesting is that, when you are not punching, you should unclench your fist.

Practically any part of the hand can be used to strike with as long as the power is applied correctly and, in addition, whilst the hand is open, you can scratch, gouge, nip, grab, pull and jab.

One word of caution I will impart is to be careful if you favour punching to the head. Remember, the reason boxing gloves were invented was not to stop the fighters from getting their faces injured, it was to protect the hands so the bloodthirsty crowds could watch longer fights. The top of the skull is exceptionally hard. Fighters were getting their knuckles broken and fights were either cut short due to swollen immobile hands, or so lacklustre as fewer and fewer punches could be thrown that the crowds were asking for their money back.

During the numerous assaults I have dealt with over the years I have met many injured assault victims, but I've also met many injured attackers. If we had an assault victim come forward who had facial injuries after being punched, one of the first things we would think of to prove that the man in the cells was involved was to get their hands photographed. Nine times out of ten their knuckles were bruised and swollen due to striking the harder parts of the skull, or they were lacerated after being caught by the victim's teeth - sometimes both.

When you consider that human saliva contains more germs and harmful bacteria than that of a dog, and there are diseases like AIDS and hepatitis around, I would be very wary about where and how I delivered a strike to an opponent's face. Unless you are a sharpshooter who can hit the end of the chin every time, I would advocate finding other ways to deliver strikes to the head and face. The heel of the palm, or the elbow, for instance. Using the heel of the palm to strike at the chin also leaves the option of raking across the eyes with the fingertips.

Incidentally, in this age of CCTV (Britain has more CCTV cameras per head of population than anywhere else in the world) when you are trying to get your point across to the police (or jury) that you were not looking for trouble and wanted a peaceful resolution to the incident, the fact that your hands are open and held in a pacifying and non-aggressive manner will help your case. This should genuinely be the case, by the way, you are a *karateka*, not a thug, and should be following the Way. I'm giving you a hint as to how to portray yourself as you really are, not providing you with a tool to help escape a conviction for assault.

Punches, when employed to the body, can be highly effective. Try them. One more thing though, keep them relaxed until the point of impact. As soon as you begin to curl your fingers inwards to make a fist, the tendons and muscles in your forearm begin to tense ever so slightly, and this increases as the fist is clenched and tightened. Any tension in your arm, no matter how slight, can slow your technique. Relax everything too, not just your clenched fist. One of the main problems I had was the relaxation of my shoulders. Once I got the hang of it my punches increased in speed and power.

When punching traditionally, with the punching hand starting from the hip, the punch begins with the palm facing upwards and it is twisted until the palm faces downwards at the point of impact. Practise leaving the wrist twist until the last possible second before impact. As you begin to practise your punches from a shorter range, this twist can augment the technique and *drill* it into the target that much more deeply.

CHAPTER TWO

The Elbow

Another much underused technique (at least in Shotokan circles), the elbow is an effective and devastating close range weapon. Probably due to the formalised ranges discussed earlier, this technique rarely, if ever, found its way into the traditional *kihon* training when I was going through the belts, yet it occurs quite often during *kata*.

As with all techniques, the best way to get a feel for the strike is by using a pad. I find focus mitts to be particularly effective for training elbow strikes like *mawashi empei*, but a kick shield is better for *yoko empei*, as the body is where that technique would be delivered.

On the subject of *mawashi empei*, I find the best way to generate impact is to try and shorten the arc which the elbow performs so that it becomes more of an "up/down" arc rather than a horizontal one. Try it, and concentrate on making the distance travelled as small as possible without losing power (a good maxim for all techniques to be honest).

Leg Techniques

Kicks can be extremely powerful, and throwing your legs all over the place in the dojo can be fun, very good for your fitness and very aesthetically pleasing. Spectacular, balletic kicks are one of the appeals of martial arts cinema, but their use in a live situation can be as dangerous for the kicker as it is for the opponent.

Kicks most certainly have their place, and, when used correctly, can be highly effective. Kicks are still part of my training regime and I suggest that you keep them in yours too. But they do come with a caveat, when it comes to live situations, so please bear in mind their limitations.

CHAPTER TWO

From the distance most fights start from (as discussed earlier) the use of head height (or even chest height for that matter) kicks is impossible. Knee strikes can be employed effectively to various areas of the legs and lower abdomen and the kick can be turned into more of a stamp against the knee or instep. So keep the distance in mind and choose the right tools for the job. The perfect distance to deliver a kick may well present itself during a fight, but don't waste your energy trying to manufacture a viable kicking distance or endanger yourself by throwing kicks in a situation where they will not work and will leave you vulnerable.

Leaving yourself vulnerable leads me nicely onto the next problem with kicks. The legs are much heavier than the arms and kicking techniques are, therefore, slower than arm techniques to deliver (at least for the majority - there is a rumour that Jet Li had to slow down when filming the kicks in *Lethal Weapon 4* because they were coming out on camera as a blur). The duration of the kick is the length of time you have to spend balanced on one leg and hence unstable.

In addition, you have to take your terrain into account. If it is a cold icy night, or the floor is covered in spilt beer and broken glass, I would be keeping both feet firmly on the ground if I could.

Anyone who has studied karate for any length of time will have found that *mawashi geri* was not always in the arsenal of kicks and, indeed, many others have been added over the years (the more spectacular spinning kicks for instance). It could be argued that these kicks emerged as a result of the tournament style of karate and the unrealistic distances which they utilise.

Originally, I believe there were only three. *Mae geri* for kicking to the front, *yoko geri* for kicking to the side, and *ushiro geri* for kicking to the rear. These are all to be delivered in the direction I have stated. Moving sideways along the *dojo* in order to deliver side kicks, and spinning round to deliver back kicks as you move forwards, lend themselves to line training. But the kicks were, in

CHAPTER TWO

my opinion, developed to cover the *karateka* through a complete circle and, depending upon where he found himself in relation to his opponent during a fight, he had a kick, or a slight variation thereof, which he could deliver in a straight line, with lots of power and very little thought about what kick to use.

They all involve the raising of the knee and the thrusting outwards of the leg in the chosen direction. They are basically the same kick. It is only the direction the foot travels that varies, and this will naturally vary the striking surface too. In the three images below, I have chosen the impact point on my opponent as the knee in keeping with the intended pragmatism of this text, but they could be employed just as well at targets both higher and lower than this.

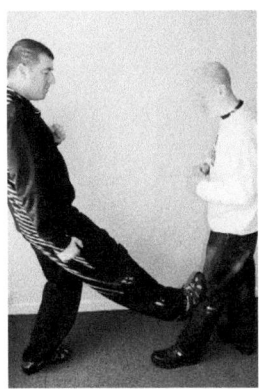
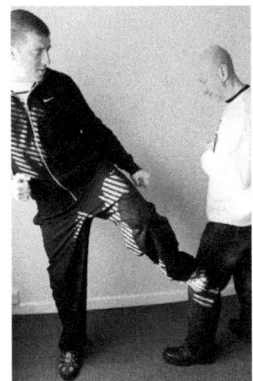
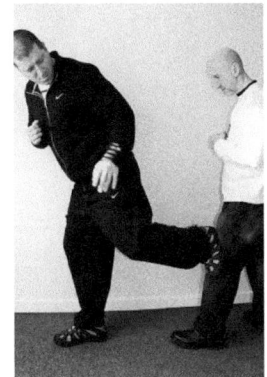

If you employ this principle, the mindset you create will negate any mental stalling you suffer as you decide which kick to use. Merely take it that you wish to drive your foot into your opponent's thigh/knee/ankle with no thought to what you should employ to accomplish it and nature will take its course.

I also think that there could be some leg techniques which have been misconstrued, either intentionally or by accident, due to increased flexibility and the employment of unrealistic distances. If you work on the maxim that historically (in karate at least), the kicks were employed as low level attacks with the legs as a primary target, could the more circular ones actually be misconstrued throws and sweeps?

Mikazuki-geri and *Ura-Mikazuki Geri,* the inside and outside crescent kicks, could actually be strikes to the inside and outside of the knee...

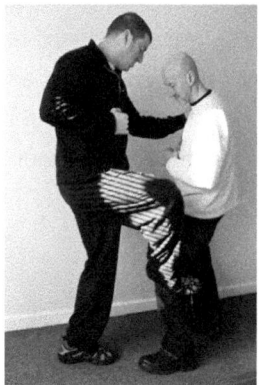 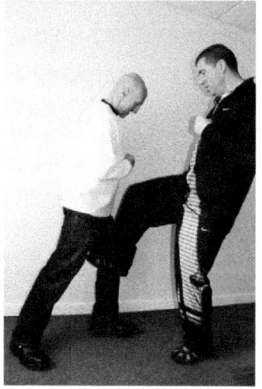

...or, at their very lowest, a means of sweeping the feet away similar to *ashi barai.*

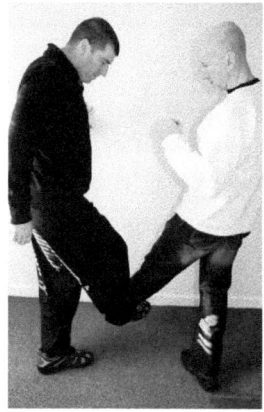 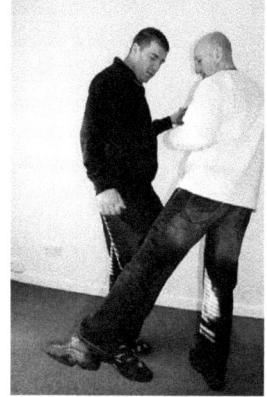

CHAPTER TWO

You only have to watch a Muay Thai match or MMA match to see the effectiveness of low level *mawashi geri,* but I can also see its value as a sweeping technique. I spent a long time, however, trying to think of a practical source for its relative, the *gyaku-mawashi geri*, sometimes known as *ushiro mawashi geri* and, in English, the hook kick. The problem was that I was looking at it as a kicking technique, when I should have looked at it in the context of a throw.

A vertical grappling scenario unfolds where you are struggling with your opponent. Utilising the principles of *hikite* described above, you managed to wrench him to one side so the majority, of not all of his bodyweight, is over one leg. You would then be free to twist your hips, bringing your far leg through as you do so, and reaping his standing leg from under him. These are the *exact* body mechanics required for *gyaku-mawashi-geri,* but employed in a different manner to execute a simple, and well known, throw.

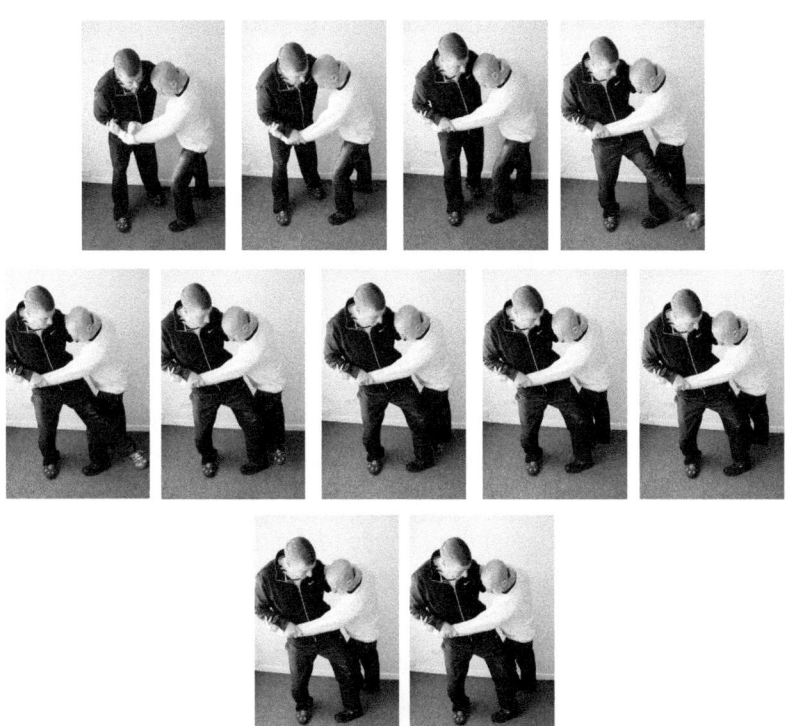

So, other than the original three kicks, the others, although known as kicks now, were more likely sweeps and throws.

Combinations

The majority of combinations practised in a traditional Shotokan *dojo* are based on the "block, then counter" scenario. As, in this instance, we are working on the premise that blocks are actually misinterpreted strikes, and the distance used in the dojo is not realistic, this renders the "block then counter" scenario somewhat defunct.

Combinations in combat sports are an effective tool, as they are generally carried out within the confines of the particular sport's guidelines and rules. This is because the reaction of the opponent is also conditioned by the same rules.

Boxers will always stay in each other's punching range, because that is where they need to be too. I have seen some really boring kickboxing matches where a "puncher" was fighting a "kicker" and they spent the entire time just trying to find their respective ranges and constantly cancelling each other out.

Now, problems with combinations arise when there are no rules binding the opponent you face. Is he a striker? A grappler? A kicker? How are you going to find out? The simple answer to this question is that you will find out by fighting him, there is no other way.

Watch an MMA match, which, although it has rules, boasts a wider variety of techniques than most other combat sports out there. Nine times out of ten you will see the fighters delivering single techniques, either to set up a takedown or to prevent themselves committing so much they are caught by one. The combinations only really come in when one of their single techniques lands effectively. The opponent staggers and then the other fighter swarms all over him or her.

When you practise combinations over and over again, your muscles "remember", so as soon as you throw the first technique of your combination, your muscles are setting up for whatever comes next. If they do this in a real situation, what are you going to do when the first attack fails? Or the first attack succeeds but the opponent does not react the way you expected?

I believe it is far better to train single techniques. There are a number of different ways to strike someone but they are all variations on a theme. The drilling of single basic straightforward strikes may seem boring until you look deeper into them.

Concentrate on the mechanics, strive to make each technique quicker and sharper than the last. Concentrate simply on getting your weapon from A to B with as little fuss and as much speed as possible. Remember the above comments regarding the three basic kicks? The same tactic could be utilised with your other weapons.

If you drill the same technique but vary angles, distances and the orientation of you to your opponent, so that they are always effective from wherever you happen to find yourself, the potentially-crippling mental processes of selecting technique can effectively be minimised.

The right tools for the job

There is much debate about whether high kicks are an effective street-fighting tool and, I have to say, no matter how flexible I was, I would always be more comfortable kicking to the knee, ankle or thigh than the chest or head, mainly because the weapon is nearer the target. Attacking the upper body with my feet when I have hands and elbows much closer is not really logical.

Think of the importance of speed and balance in conflict. If the body mechanics are right, weapons do not have to wind up and travel great distances to be effective. The shorter your technique's travelling time, the less time the opponent has to prepare or take evasive action. It stands to reason then that you should use the legs to attack the lower body and the hands and arms to attack the upper.

CHAPTER TWO

I know there are people out there who have lightning-fast high kicks which they can deliver with a hell of a lot of power and fair play to them. I am speaking, however, from a pragmatic standpoint. During a real, violent encounter, would you drop to one knee and deliver a punch to someone's thigh? You would not. Yet in some areas the debate still rages about whether a head height kick is the way to go.

In addition, the use of kicks to the lower body does not require any warm up. In the dojo, get as flexible as you can, warm up and throw those high kicks as high as you wish, because this will mean that even whilst you are cold, your muscles are longer and more relaxed than average and the power in your low kicks will be augmented by that.

I have mentioned elbows and knees as well as punches and kicks during this section, but what about a head butt? The purists are probably screaming at me now, but I am afraid they are right there in your arsenal.

In the *Gojushiho kata*, there is a technique whereby the *karateka* extends both their hands out at shoulder height, and then whips them around to the rear, leaning forward slightly as they do so. I cannot see how this can be effective as a double punch to the kidneys of an opponent who has you in a bear hug from behind, as I have heard it described. The technique executed in this manner has no power and is completely impractical. No - the technique makes much more sense if you see it as grabbing someone by the shoulders and then pulling them sharply into a descending headbutt.

Impact training

Even if you cannot do it all the time, you must, at some point in your karate training, learn what it is like to strike something other than fresh air. Whether you use a *makiwara*, a heavy bag, focus mitts or a kick shield, experiencing the sensation of a technique impacting

CHAPTER TWO

against a surface is essential. You will find that your technique changes, not substantially, but there will be minor alterations you will make and they will make your techniques that much more effective.

One caveat, however, is that the changes you make to deliver the technique into the pad more effectively may not translate to delivering the techniques into fresh air. If you watch a Muay Thai practitioner, for instance, the roundhouse kicks he throws into fresh air cause him to spin on the spot because he is used to driving the power through a pad. The way some Shotokan techniques are practised, particularly kicks, do not tend to lend themselves to this and damage to joints could occur unless care is taken.

Chapter 3

Anatomy and strategy

So, when performing our techniques now, we are moving with more freedom and the flowery, extraneous movements of our techniques have been cropped. Our karate is already looking leaner and meaner but to increase its effectiveness even more we need to discuss targets.

In the old days, when karate was being studied on Okinawa and was not a worldwide commercial success, much emphasis was placed upon the vital points of the body and how (and even when) to strike them. *The Bible of Karate – Bubishi* translated with commentary by Patrick McCarthy and published by Charles E. Tuttle Company, Inc. (1995) is an excellent in-depth view of the more pragmatic side of *karatedo* and I would urge readers to seek it out (if you haven't already).

I am in no way intending to plagiarise this work but, as the majority of vital points are all well known anyway, I intend to conduct a short tour around the human body and discuss certain sensitive areas and the best weapons for targeting them.

When training in traditional karate, one of the first things that you become familiar with are the three areas the body is generally split into, those being *jodan*, for the head, *chudan*, for the torso and *gedan* for everything below the waist.

When conducting formalised sparring where you would name

your target in order that the opponent could practise his blocking techniques, these three areas were the ones you named. For the purposes of learning to "block" techniques (remember: they are not blocks), this is adequate as the opponent knows the general area the technique will be aimed at and can take appropriate action, but from the point of view of the attacker, it is impossibly vague.

The head (Jodan)

Practically speaking, this is the fighter's favourite area to target. Whether this is derived from a desire to seek the knockout or the fact that the injuries caused are so much more visible, and therefore more demoralising is a matter of debate, but the fact remains that when a fight starts outside, the majority of strikes thrown are to the region of the head.

The cranium, at the very top of the head, consists of bones which have fused as a person has grown into adulthood. It is there to protect the brain from impact. As such, it is extremely dense and resilient and, although a heavy percussive blow can cause some damage to an opponent, I would be tempted to remove this from the list of viable targets an unarmed fighter should attack due to the high risk of self injury.

The forehead is also a dense sheet of bone designed to protect our highly developed frontal lobe. It is also the impact point for the delivery of a headbutt, which demonstrates its resilience. It does however have a flaw. It is probably the furthest point from the neck on the head, so a good driving blow straight at the forehead can cause a whiplash effect strong enough to render an opponent unconscious by shaking the brain in the skull. (Warning: anything which attacks the neck or spine, directly or indirectly, can cause permanent damage and sometimes death. You must be justified in any strike you use (more on the legal ramifications later).

The recommended weapon for striking this area would be the

CHAPTER THREE

heel of the palm. This area of the hand is quite fleshy and would be protected from the hard bones in the forehead. Use of the fist to strike this area may have the desired effect, but would more likely result in a set of busted knuckles.

The eyes are an obvious vulnerable point, but are not as easy to target from a striking point of view as you would expect. I would not advocate use of *ippon* or *nihon nukite* in a live scenario as the eyes are extremely small targets surrounded by hard bone.

The best way to attack the eyes from a striking point of view would be the use of a *mawashi empei* to the orbit, that's the ridge of bone that encircles the eye socket. It fractures a little more easily than the rest of the skull as it is weaker due to the fact that it surrounds an opening and, if you have ever had yours fractured or seen someone else after they had theirs done, the swelling is rapid and wince-inducing. The other way to attack the eyes is obviously during a grappling scenario, where a gouge can be employed.

The nose comprises a protruding bone from the skull, which terminates at the bridge and is thereafter replaced by a length of cartilage. There has been much debate over the years as to whether it is possible to dislodge this cartilage and send it upwards, like a missile, into the brain. I honestly have no idea whether it would or not, but I would certainly not like to be the first test case in court if it were true. But a good blow to the nose can cause it to bleed and make the eyes water, making it a sound distraction technique either to set up a further technique or to get away.

If the nose is "broken", which usually means the cartilage being dislodged from the bone or snapped, it can also interrupt their breathing. My recommended weapon would be the heel of the palm once again, the elbow (as in a *mawashi empei*) or a hammer fist (*tettsui*). You can also use your forehead, but be prepared to see a few stars yourself if your aim is off!

Although it has been proven time and time again that a solid blow from a fist can do the damage, opponents have an annoying

CHAPTER THREE

habit of moving about. Should you miss, once again, the knuckles would not withstand impact to the skull. (The nose can also be manipulated in a grappling scenario, if the fingers are forced into the nostrils and then pulled away from the face... well, you can imagine, but it would not be pretty and it would be extremely painful, both at the time and afterwards, for the unlucky recipient.)

The philthrum is on the top lip, at the centre, directly below the nose. It is very painful to be struck here but it is a target that is not that easy to get at. The best method would be in the scenario described for the execution of *shuto uke*, where it could be struck or used as a fulcrum to lever the head back and interrupt balance. It is also a favoured striking point for *ippon ken* (the one knuckle fist in traditional Okinawan karate), a technique which causes a lot of pain with little effort).

The point of the chin, called the "sweet spot" by Mohammed Ali, is the optimum point to strike an opponent if you want to knock them out. As with the forehead, a good solid strike to this area can shake the brain within the skull and thereby cause unconsciousness. Most people are surprised the first time they manage to hit this spot right, as it feels like you hardly touched your opponent at all. This is because if you get the angle right, the strike catches the chin at just the right angle to spin the head and shake the brain, not break the bone. Once again, the fist is usually employed for this, but you could also use the elbow or the heel of the palm for the same effect.

The throat is probably the weakest point on the human body. It has never evolved since before we walked upright. If you were on all fours it would be protected merely by being underneath your body, but now we walk upright the entire trachea is exposed from the base of the head to the juncture of the clavicle. A solid strike anywhere along the length of this can result in serious injury or death.

I cannot stress how much a strike to this area really must be a last resort. From a grappling point of view, attacking the throat is

CHAPTER THREE

still dangerous, but the degree of pressure and angle of attack can be managed more effectively. Digging the thumb in on one side of the trachea and the fingers in on the other and squeezing is an extremely effective choke hold, but care must be taken that the trachea is not dislodged. Pushing from the front with the forearm can elicit a backwards lean and a breaking of grip by your opponent and, from the rear, a choke hold with the forearm across the trachea can stop the opponent drawing breath.

At the base of the trachea, where your clavicle bones meet, is a U-shaped notch nicknamed the "jugular notch". If you push this area with one or two fingers it causes an extremely uncomfortable sensation for the opponent, driving them backwards and causing an involuntary dropping of the chin towards the chest. This used to be in the police self defence manual but it was removed due to the health implications inherent in attacking the throat.

So ironically, although the throat is probably the weakest spot on the body and is not that difficult to land an effective technique on, it must be avoided unless absolutely necessary because of its vulnerability.

The mandible, or lower jaw is weakest where it meets the skull. This is the only joint in the head area (not counting the flexibility of the upper vertebrae) and this makes it a weak spot in itself. A solid strike can break or dislocate the jaw at this point because it is where the jaw bone tapers before joining the skull.

A strike anywhere along the jawline is also capable of knocking out an opponent, but obviously the solidity of the impact must increase the closer to the skull the blow lands. I would advocate, once again, the use of the elbow or the heel of the palm for this strike as minimal movement by an opponent can result in a missed strike and damage to a clenched fist.

The temple is a natural recess in the skull just behind the orbit of the eye sockets. If the cranium has a weak spot, this is it. It may be inadvertently struck by a badly-aimed strike seeking the orbit and was a favoured target for *hiraken* when I was young.

CHAPTER THREE

It must be stressed, once again, that this is a weak spot in an area of bone designed to protect the brain, so, whilst I can tell you that *hiraken* or *mawashi empei* are both viable weapons for this spot, it is best avoided unless absolutely necessary.

The ear is, like the nose, largely composed of cartilage and, also like the nose, is favoured as an area ripe for biting in a last-resort scenario as it can cause debilitating pain to be bitten in the ear and it does not take much to bite off a portion, a serious psychological advantage in a last resort situation. The best method of attack for the ears is a slap, either with the hand flat or slightly cupped. This causes air to be forced down the ear canal, resulting in a feeling of compression in that area, serious ringing in the ears and, in some cases, rupture of the tympanum. All our balance is centred in the fluid within the ear and a solid strike as described can seriously compromise an opponent's balance. In addition, as the ears protrude from the side of the head, pulling and twisting them can greatly assist in a grappling scenario.

The "mandibular angle" is a nerve cluster seated in a recess directly below the ear and behind the vertical section of the mandible. It is best found by forcing the tip of the thumb into the recess and pushing hard inwards and upwards. It will cause the opponent to lean his head away so a firm hand on the other side of the head to hold him in place is sometimes necessary.

Further down the neck, along the same line, the nerve travels under the sterno-cleido mastoid muscle (that thick band of muscle that runs up the side of your neck). If you drive the tip of your thumb into this muscle with the feeling that you want to force the fibres of the muscle out of the way, then twist, it tweaks the nerves and causes a jolt of intense pain.

I will be mentioning some more pressure points as we progress, so it is probably timely for me to mention their downside. Firstly, they do not work on everybody. It is a scientific fact that pressure points differ between races, and I have also met people of the same

CHAPTER THREE

ethnicity who have differing reactions. One was writhing in agony, the other looked at me nonplussed. Be prepared for them to fail.

Also, the pain caused by tweaking a pressure point does not increase the longer you hold it on, and is gone as soon as you release. They are best used as quick fixes to gain the upper hand just long enough to do what you need to do. They are also extraordinarily difficult to target on a moving opponent, though they are highly effective when seeking advantage in a grappling situation.

The carotid artery is also protected by the aforementioned sterno-cleido mastoid muscle and feeds blood to the brain. When you see someone falling asleep having been held in a rear naked choke during an MMA match, it is due to the blood supply to the brain being cut off by the pincer-like attack of the arm when the biceps presses on one side of the neck and the forearm presses on the other. It does not take long for the squeeze to take effect and care must be taken, as the longer the brain is deprived of oxygenated blood the greater the risk of brain damage and death.

The back of the neck is usually only presented as a viable target if an opponent bends at the waist as he comes in at you. Once again, this is very much a last resort scenario (there is a reason why "rabbit punches" are not allowed in boxing) as the most viable weapon for this is a downwards *empei*. The muscles at the back of the neck may be dense, but they are protecting the spine, and damage to the spine can be life changing, if not life ending.

Did you notice that, on our tour of the head, there were a lot of places where it was dangerous to hit and none which were ideally attacked with the fist? I know I have mentioned it before, but it bears repeating - keep your hands open, they are far more versatile that way.

If you are a dyed in the wool puncher, worry not, there will be plenty of opportunities for you to ply your trade as we work our way down the body.

CHAPTER THREE

The torso (Chudan)

For our purposes this will also include the arms.

The majority of sensitive areas are on the front of the body. This is most likely due to the fact that our body design began to evolve before we walked upright. The organs are protected to some degree by slabs of muscle and the flexible cage of ribs, but there are areas where there are chinks in the armour so to speak, and some of the areas we discuss will be exploiting these.

The trapezius muscles are the sloping muscles that run from the base of the neck along the rear of each shoulder and actually extend some way down the back. They are quite thick, dense areas, particularly at the top of the shoulder and a solid hammer fist (*tettsui*) or *empei* can upset the balance, as can a double strike to both shoulders simultaneously, which can send your opponent to the ground.

The limiting factor in attacking the trapezius muscles is that they are most effectively tackled from behind. Should you need to break the grip of an opponent on an ally, striking this muscle in the first instance is an effective choice.

The clavicles, or collar bones are the "shock absorbers" for the shoulders. They keep everything in place and are usually the first thing to snap or dislocate when someone tries to break their fall, thereby protecting the rest of the structure. They are not an easy area to target with a strike, as when someone "bunches" up ready for conflict they are pushed below and behind muscle. If you do try to strike them, however, I recommend the heel of the palm, which can have the effect of interrupting rhythm on one of those rare occasions that you see a haymaker coming. There is also a nerve cluster behind the clavicle, which is extremely difficult to target from the front but, once again, can be targeted from the rear in a vertical grappling scenario or when assisting an ally. It is best accessed by grabbing the clavicle and pushing the fingers down behind it.

CHAPTER THREE

The same warning goes with this pressure point as all the others. I have seen people that it does not work on, so if are going to try it, have a contingency plan in place, just in case.

The shoulder is an extremely mobile ball-and-socket joint protected by a dense deltoid muscle but, as is so often the case in nature, if you go to the other side of the structure, you will find it is not very protected at all. The armpit, whilst a somewhat unsavoury area on some, is shielded by the deltoids, pectoralis and latissimus dorsi. If you should get the chance, a solid punch into the hollow between these muscle groups can be debilitating and painful.

On the inside of the upper arm there is a small gap in between your biceps and triceps. If you push your fingers into this gap on your own arm you will feel a tingling, twanging sensation as far down your arm as your fingers. Once again, where there's armour on one side there's vulnerability on the other. It is not an easy place to hit (although I once saw someone take a punch on that area by accident and it had the effect of "deadening" his entire arm, so it is viable if you are a good shot). Digging the fingers into it in a grappling scenario can prove quite effective, as can a strike from the forearm.

The elbow joint can be used to execute an arm bar, as seen earlier, or can be hyper-extended through striking the back of the joint when the arm is locked straight. This is extremely painful and can cause long-term damage to the unlucky victim. As with all joint work, care should be taken when practising techniques but it is worth spending time finding ways to manipulate joints and their strengths and weaknesses.

The same nerve we referred to in the neck runs down the arm and then around the forearm and is hidden under the dense muscle that tenses and raises itself when you tightly clench your fist. It is possible to dig your thumb into this muscle and deliver a substantial amount of pain, but it does take considerable grip strength. I have found attacking this area most effective through utilising a hammer

CHAPTER THREE

fist (*tettsui*) or merely by dropping the forearm onto it. Striking this area causes a temporary motor dysfunction. It causes the elbow to drop, the shoulder to open and, due to the slight "whiplash" effect, the head to tilt away, exposing any number of targets.

The wrist joint itself is well worth spending some time experimenting with. There is a reason why it gets priority in *taiho jutsu* and arts like *aikido*. If you can control the wrist effectively, you can manipulate the entire body.

Although there are a number of ways to gain control of the wrist, the most favoured one is for the fingers to wrap around the joint and the thumb to push into the back of the hand.

The back of the hand may not seem like a viable target, but it is another area where *ippon ken* (the one knuckle fist) can come into its own. It takes surprisingly little power to inflict pain with this strike to the back of the hand.

The fingers, when used together, can be formidable, but individually, they cannot stand the combined strength of all of yours at once. When breaking a grip (I would advocate the use of a strike elsewhere on the body to serve as a "distraction" first or you may find yourself being hit whilst trying to break the grip), attack the little finger first as that is the weak point of the clenched fist. Another excruciating attack on the fingers is to pull them apart.

Now we return to the torso. The sternum, or breastbone, is a solid length of bone running down the centre of the upper chest. It protects the heart and lungs and holds the front of the ribcage together. A solid punch to this area or, if you find yourself sideways on or attacked from behind, an *empei*, can "wind" your opponent and be a very debilitating strike.

The pectoralis or chest muscles are there to protect the upper organs of the body too, but solid strikes with fist or elbow to this region can also have the desired effect. In addition, on women, a strike to the breasts can be extremely painful (so I am reliably informed).

The heart is hidden behind the pectoralis and the sternum and,

CHAPTER THREE

whilst pinpoint accuracy is often lacking in stressful situations, a solid blow to where you *think* the heart may be would be enough. During the making of *Rocky IV*, rumour has it, Sylvester Stallone was forced to "rest" for a few days when Dolph Lundgren bruised his heart when they were sparring, so it apparently does work.

The solar plexus can be found under the "v" shaped lower edge of the ribcage. Once again, the fist and elbow are viable weapons as are (now we are getting lower) the knees. In fact, if you rotate your fist slightly, you will see that if fits quite snugly into the area in question.

A *tai chi sifu* once told me that a hard strike to the solar plexus can seriously interrupt the rhythm of the heart and have serious consequences. I cannot comment on the veracity of this claim, but I can say that being hit in this area can cause a spasm in the lungs (being "winded") which momentarily prevents you from breathing in and has brought the biggest of men to their knees. Knockouts have actually been scored in combat sports from shots hitting this area. At the very least, it renders your opponent momentarily defenceless.

The floating ribs are so called because, whilst they are secured at the rear, to the spine, they are unsecured, or "floating" on the front of the torso. Once again, fists, elbows and knees are viable weapons. In addition, on the right side, just beneath and behind the floating ribs, is the liver. A solid strike to this organ can be very painful indeed.

The abdomen is protected by muscles that are more like sheets than bunches (such as, for instance, the deltoid). If you have ever seen an abdominal cavity (not necessarily in real life, a good anatomy book will do!) you will see that the organs and intestines are neatly arranged inside with not much room to spare at all. This is why a solid strike to the abdominal wall can be so painful. No matter where it is struck, if the strike is hard enough, there is something relatively sensitive and important to the function of the human body nestling underneath. Again, fists, elbows, knees and, in some instances when opportunity knocks, the feet, are all good for this area.

On the rear of the body we have the spine. Unless you are truly in fear for your life and you have absolutely no other option *do not strike this area*. Although surrounded by robust muscle throughout the back, a solid penetrative blow can have life altering consequences (for both parties).

The kidneys sit either side of the lumbar region of the spine. As with the abdominal wall, the muscles in the lower back are like sheets and strikes to this area can easily be transmitted to the organs beneath. As with blows to the liver and the general area of the abdominal wall, there is always the risk that organs may be damaged if the blows are powerful enough. (We will talk about reasonable force later).

The lower body (Gedan)

Although I have rarely seen it done in a real scenario, attacking the lower body can be extremely effective in a live situation. It is a good area to attack with the legs as they do not have to travel far, do not lose power fighting against gravity, it takes little or no flexibility to use them and balance can be easily maintained.

The genitalia and pubic bone are a favourite point of attack. Surprisingly, I have suffered both full on strikes and glancing blows to this area and it was always that latter that hurt the most, although I have no idea why.

Even if the chosen strike misses the main target, a blow to the lower abdomen can still be debilitating (you may find, in a live situation, that the genitalia are not as easy to hit as you would think). Knees, feet and strikes with the palm or the edge of the hand are all viable. Dispel any notion that grabbing them is a good idea as clothing may get in the way.

CHAPTER THREE

This pain factor is not merely to the male of the species either, a solid strike to the pubic bone on a woman is agony (again, so I am reliably informed). The area around the genitals, the upper part of the inner thigh and through towards the anus have soft skin (another weak point caused by us walking upright when we should be on all fours) and the nerves are close to the surface, so don't worry if your aim is off, the chances are you will still get the desired effect.

The outside of the quadriceps protects a nerve cluster, the striking of which can cause what is colloquially known as a "dead leg". As well as being painful, blows to this area also cause an involuntary sensory motor dysfunction, so even if your opponent is feeling no pain, a blow to this area can still render his leg useless. The knees or shins (utilising *mawashi geri*) are the chosen weapons for this area. As long as the body mechanics are correct, a knee strike to this area takes very little effort and is extremely fast to deliver. In a vertical grappling scenario, your opponent will also be blind to it.

The inside of the thigh, whilst not immediately apparent as a viable target, is an excellent spot to aim for with a short sharp kick using the instep as the area of impact (this kick is used in Kyokushin). It takes little or no time to deliver and can seriously upset the balance of your opponent.

The knee joint cannot be overemphasised as a viable target for bringing someone down. Patrick Swayze espoused its benefits in *Roadhouse* (the uncut version now available on DVD, for some reason all the strikes to the knee were removed from the VHS version) and he was absolutely right. *Mawashi geri* or *yoko geri* to either the inside or outside, or a *mae geri* to the patella, which causes an extremely painful hyperextension of the joint (see the earlier section), are all suitable. They would be an especially attractive target if the opponent was big and heavy (whether this is caused by fat or muscle does not matter) because the knees bear a lot of weight and no matter how strong a man makes his thighs or calves, they both end at the knee. It would be very easy to cause damage to this joint, so please take care in training (in fact, when attacking each other with this technique, never do it without a kick shield in the way and make sure the person holding the pad is ready and can brace for impact).

The gastrocnemius (the calf muscle) also protects a nerve cluster and a strike to that area (with the heel, for instance) can break an opponent's balance. It can also be hit with a *mawashi geri* if desired.

The good thing about all the pressure points on the limbs is that the strikes do not have to be pin point accurate. Any blow to the general area will do and there is little chance of damaging your own weapons should you err from the target.

The shin bone is a particularly good target if you wear hard soled shoes. Although practitioners of Muay Thai have the hardest shins in the world, lots of people do not and there are many nerves near the surface. A hard sole kicked into the shin, or, if you were grabbed from behind, the heel run down the shin, can be very painful indeed.

The ankle is another joint vulnerable to attack from the side, although not as easily accessible as the knee. A stamping *fumakomi,* if viable at the time, would do the trick, but the ankle is weakest when it is swept, taking the feet out from under your opponent. Although all practitioners of traditional karate should be familiar with *ashi-barai* (the foot sweep), do not underestimate, nor neglect, the use of a low *mawashi geri* to this area either.

Finally, the foot is a relatively flat area of skin and muscle filled with small metatarsal bones which can be very easily damaged by stamping, although footwear would afford the foot some degree of protection.

So, whilst the above list is extensive, it is by no means exhaustive and I might well have missed out areas on the body which have worked particularly well for you. My reasons for taking the time to run through these points is that, as a pragmatic *karateka*, the concept of merely aiming for *jodan, chudan* or *gedan* is too vague and targeting specific areas should be your aim, (no pun intended).

Learning about the human body and its weaknesses, what weapons to attack the various areas with and the possible ramifications of doing so must be included in any realistic training session. It would be outrageously remiss of any instructor to fail to educate their students in the specifics of the potential injuries caused, and to educate them in how to hit the body without injuring themselves.

Strategy

As can be seen from the section above, there is a host of different available targets and even more means of attacking them. If you were ever unfortunate enough to need to use them outside, you could easily be so confused as to what to do that while you were thinking you became a sitting duck. As I stated earlier, I am not a fan of learning combinations as factors come into play during a real encounter which do not exist in a sterile dojo environment, and I would always favour the drilling of single techniques *ad nauseam* so that they become entrenched in your muscle memory.

Over the years lots of texts have mentioned limiting the number of techniques you practise to cut down on your choices and thereby free your mind. I do think this is an excellent idea, but it was always at the back of my mind: What would I do if my favoured attack failed?

I recognise the importance of, and am a big fan of *kata*. As well as learning the *bunkai,* which is the pinnacle of pragmatic karate, they are an excellent means of retaining agility, flexibility, strength and focus. But I do not see them as a series of combinations; I see them as a collection of a past master's favourite *single* techniques, put together into a *kata* for future generations to learn.

You will notice, if you practice a *kata* long enough, that there are usually recurring themes within them (I mentioned the high

CHAPTER THREE

incidence of *shuto* in *Kanku dai* earlier). This is because they recognised the importance of a personal fighting style which suited your body type and had techniques which you found easy to execute.

This is why I think it is worth spending some time analysing your personal fighting style. What techniques do you favour? Which do you seem best suited to performing? What targets are you aiming for? What are the best ways, using your favourite techniques, to end a fight as quickly as possible?

You also need to decide which of your techniques will work on any person, regardless of size or gender, so that you are not intimidated by persons larger than you, and, just as important, do not underestimate people who are smaller than you.

You will probably find, if you are being realistic, that it is the simple, sometimes more brutal and less attractive techniques that seem to work in a live situation.

Do not limit your attacks to one area. Think of your opponent's body as a machine, if you break one part, if has an effect on all the others.

Do you ruin his balance when you attack? Affect his senses? His ability to breathe (momentarily of course)? These are the effects which, when inflicted, are more likely to work and to end the fight. People fight one-armed and they fight through pain, sometimes with broken limbs. Some people have an iron chin. Your opponent may be under the influence of some substance (either legal or illegal) which means you cannot rely on inflicting pain in the normal way. Your techniques need to work regardless of mental state and stature.

By fitting your favoured techniques to areas on your opponent's body which will have these effects, you maximise your chances of success. Thus, your personal fighting strategy is borne not just from the utilisation of anatomy, but from what you hold in your personal arsenal, so that the technique you use is never wasted.

CHAPTER THREE

Tai sabaki

So what of the defender - the *uke*, who receives the technique on the other side of the sparring partnership? As I have already advised that blocks are potentially misunderstood as such, this renders the traditional methods of halting the attacks defunct.

This is where the facet of karate known as *tai-sabaki* comes into play - the movement and positioning of your body in order for you to effectively avoid the attack from your opponent and place yourself in an advantageous position either to run away or attack your attacker (for a realistic training scenario, both options should be practised). With a little practice, movement can become fluid and instinctive. It is worth practising movement in different directions to ascertain where you emerge in relation to your opponent and what strikes in your personal bank of techniques can be used from these positions. (Remember the maintenance of balance as you move.)

When beginners learn *kumite*, particularly in Shotokan, the attacks are linear and the *uke* moves along the same line as his attacker. This unfortunately creates the mindset that you should stay in your attacker's line of fire and rely on your blocks until an opening presents itself. Under the formal training distances employed in some dojo, this is a relatively easy and safe thing to do. Use of *tai sabaki* at these distances can sometimes be intercepted, as the attacker has time to readjust. Close the distance, as discussed earlier, however, and the simple effectiveness of diagonal movements to place yourself outside the line of attack and set up an attack or escape of your own reveals itself.

The attacker should not be rigid. He should deliver his attack but not freeze at the culmination of its delivery. If *tai-sabaki* is employed effectively, the defender should no longer be there anyway and the robotic back and forth of formal traditional sparring would regain more of its fluidity and vitality.

CHAPTER THREE

A matter which I intend to discuss in detail a little later is that of the pre-emptive strike. In a formal sparring scenario, could you actually beat the attacker to the punch (literally)? Theoretically, if you move as soon as you see your attacker move, rather than waiting for the arm or leg to extend so you can deal with that, could you employ a fast, linear technique to interrupt their forward movement and disrupt the attack?

A great deal of benefit can be gained for both parties utilising this kind of scenario and it can bring a little healthy competition to a training situation, but utilisation of control in sparring and dojo work is paramount and, bearing this in mind, great care must be taken with this method. Padding and protective equipment for these kind of exercises is a necessity.

Chapter 4

Going to the ground

Fighting on the ground has been elevated to an art form all on its own. The Gracie family raised the bar and created an entire system of controlling and submitting an opponent on the ground. This has won and lost belts in the MMA world and it has reached the point where, if you do not have a ground game in MMA, sooner or later you are going to come unstuck.

The ground, however, is the last place you want to be in a real situation. The floor of the Octagon is nice and clean (maybe a little bloodstained if you are later in the fight card). There is a referee to watch over you and ensure that the techniques used fall into the set of rules which helped to bring MMA from the backstreets to the forefront and, if you or your opponent are not working hard enough, or are not advancing your position, he will stand you up, separate you and let you start again.

In the real world, you go to the ground and suddenly find yourself on a concrete floor with broken glass, spilt fluids and dirty needles littered across it. It has been raining and the recess which would be invisible on a dry day is now a deep puddle. There is no referee, but there are several onlookers who will stick a boot in your face if the opportunity arises, and your opponent has probably got some friends who will be more than willing to throw a few kicks your way. The assault upon you, should they gain the upper hand, will not stop

CHAPTER FOUR

because a buzzer sounds, and it will not stop when a referee steps in. It will stop when your attackers' hands and feet are too sore to continue, or they are out of breath.

From a policing point of view, the main objective is to restrain your opponent so you can get the cuffs on him (I joined before the use of CS and PAVA came in and we had chain link cuffs and a truncheon) so we were taught holds on the ground to render our opponents immobile. The holds came from *Taiho-jutsu* via Judo, where there is a ground game element. The problem with restraining your opponent in a scarf hold or an arm bar, however, is that you would have to be on the ground too.

In an arena or an octagon, that is fine. Both fighters can afford to be patient, work their positions and try for a submission. They have the luxury of knowing what their opponent will and will not do to them within certain parameters.

When I talk about going to the ground I am not necessarily saying that you could be the victim of a throw or strike, though that could happen. There is the environment to take into account also. Is it wet and slippery? Is the ground frozen? Are there imperfections in the surface you are fighting on which could trip or unbalance the unwary fighter?

One of the things a lot of traditional martial artists have mentioned over the years is the big difference between sterile training and real confrontation. I am not just thinking of the mental element (more on that later), but how potentially *messy* things are outside. Overly complicated techniques that have been drilled to the extreme in the dojo are suddenly impossible to execute because of the effects of adrenalin (the main reason techniques should be streamlined, not flowery) and, more importantly your opponent is not your fellow *karateka* who you have known and trained with for years. Your opponent has an unknown skill set and will not react the way you think he will.

From a ground fighting point of view, if you were to execute a reaping throw similar to the one I discussed in the section on kicks and your opponent were a *judoka* or similar, he would be confident that he could break his fall and would let himself drop. You would probably have your hands full if you followed him down and a stalemate would probably be reached if you remain standing, which is fine, because you can get away now. (Ego has no part in survival. Much more on ego later.)

Now, if your opponent is a striker, whose comfort zone and element is the use of techniques whilst standing, or a street fighter (who just watched his one favourite technique fail on you and is now out of ideas), and you were to execute the same reaping throw, his reaction could be far more visceral.

No-one likes to fall. It is one of the strange things again that links back to us walking upright. Our balance is off compared to our four-legged ancestors and can be manipulated. Losing your balance can cause involuntary movements, like putting out your hands, even though you know that you would do yourself more damage by doing so. I have seen drunk people take some amazing dives and look as if they are going to need a visit to a hospital, but they jumped up, dusted themselves off and carried on. They would probably have a few bruises and aches the next morning which they could not account for, but because their drunkenness relaxed them, when they fell, they escaped serious injury.

People who practise the grappling arts like Judo are taught how to break their fall before anything else. This is because, once we pass the stage of baby relaxation and have felt the pain of falling a few times, our first instinct when we begin to fall is to tense ready for the impact, and this is precisely the opposite of what is required. We are so keen to stay on our feet that falling creates a deep-seated fundamental fear which must be overridden.

Going back to our striking opponent then, if you are in a vertical grappling scenario when you take his legs, he will panic. It may be on a deep, subconscious level but the panic will still be there, and

CHAPTER FOUR

his body will tense. If he has hold of you when that involuntary tensing occurs, his grip will tighten exponentially and he will drag you down with him - not from any combat perspective, but from a deep-rooted instinct to arrest his own descent.

If you should go to the ground, your main objective is to disengage from your opponent and get back to your feet as soon as possible.

Now, techniques which serve you well standing may not be so good when you hit the ground, because the proper use of body mechanics for the application of power is not available. My advice, should you ever find yourself in this position, is to attack soft tissue.

Do not think about breaking your opponent's grip by manipulating their fingers, because whilst they are holding you they have one less weapon to strike you with. Remember that his movement is now impaired just as much as yours and he does not have the evasive options available when standing. Jabbing and gouging the eyes, twisting the ears, slapping the ears, biting the nose (provided you are not too concerned about infection) are all viable options which can be effectively resorted to with minimum movement and minimum power but can be excruciating for the opponent.

Please understand, I am not advocating that gouging out someone's eye is a main objective when on the ground. You are trying to facilitate the breaking of your opponent's grip as you are in danger there. Once they release you, disengage and stand back up, either to press the advantage if you have no way of escaping or to run away if you have.

With the advent of MMA, the chances of encountering an opponent who has some knowledge of the ground game are much higher. But there is a caveat to learning the MMA techniques, and this is advice for people who practice MMA as well as people who may find themselves in a fight against them. Your ground game may be devastating, but it is still governed by a set of rules. When you engage in an MMA match, or ground fighting in a judo dojo for that

CHAPTER FOUR

matter, attacks to soft tissue with fingers and open hands are banned. *They are not banned outside.* In a combat sport, if techniques are banned, you do not have to plan to defend yourself against them. A boxer does not work on defence against kicks, MMA fighters do not learn to defend against small joint manipulation, head butts, finger jabs and gouges, judoka do not learn to defend against strikes (at least the majority no longer do, although they used to).

People who know how to handle themselves on the floor are not to be taken lightly, rules or not. They can swarm all over you and choke you out before you even realise you have gone down.

In order for your karate to be pragmatic, you must spend at least some of your training time on groundwork. Learn how to fall, learn restraints (you never know when they could come in handy).

There is no safe way to practice attacking the soft tissue. If you practise to "just miss" (a common fault in some dojo) that is how you would fight, and you would "just miss" his eyes when you really needed to hit them.

Spend some time grappling on the ground, but start from standing, as though the fight has taken you there, and make yourself at least comfortable in that environment so that, should you be unfortunate enough to go down, the arena will not be so alien that you will freeze.

And always remember, your objective is to disengage and get back up as quickly as possible.

(N.B I would strongly recommend Geoff Thompson's series of books on ground fighting and Iain Abernathy's "Throws for Strikers" for further reading. See the bibliography for more details).

Ground fighting and traditional karate

No book on pragmatic fighting can really be called comprehensive unless it includes fighting on the ground, but this is about making

CHAPTER FOUR

traditional karate training more streetwise. When I first thought of including ground fighting in this text, I wondered if it was a complete departure from the art and I was adding elements.

This clearly flies in the face of what I am trying to achieve. To *add* an element of combat into the mix implies that the core art is deficient in some way. I therefore returned to the original question which gave rise to my writing this: What did Funakoshi change to make the art more palatable to the Japanese?

Karate, on Okinawa, was (and is) a civilian fighting system based on actual combat. The sporting element did not come until much later (if what I have read is true, Funakoshi was not too keen on the sporting element, rather he wanted it to be a spiritual endeavour). In order for their art to be effective, it had to cover all aspects, and I am sure that the original *karateka* would have given the same consideration to going to the ground as we do.

Although *kata bunkai* falls outside the scope of this book, I would advise the *karateka* to look at the *kata* from a ground fighting perspective. I have already mentioned the last move in, *Hangetsu*. This could just as easily be demonstrative of an arm bar on the ground, as could the technique immediately after the jump in *Heian Godan*.

I believe ground fighting has always been there, but it has been hidden or intentionally misinterpreted. The obvious question is - why? To answer this, I decided to try and look at it from Master Funakoshi's point of view.

You come from a small annexed island with what is seen by the Japanese watching it as a quaint indigenous art and try to "sell" it to those who have a long and justifiably proud history of *Bushido*. What can you offer that is different?

The main unarmed disciplines favoured by your potential customers are sumo, aikido and ju-jitsu, the latter having recently been formulated into the hugely popular Judo by Jigoro Kano. It is a well known fact that Funakoshi and Kano were friends. Indeed, the idea for the *gi* and coloured belt system used in karate came from Kano's Judo. It would be folly to turn up on Japanese soil and try to sell them an art containing grappling and ground fighting when they are already well versed in it anyway. It would be far more advisable to "re-interpret" such techniques from a striking perspective, and a safe striking perspective at that, considering the fact that he ultimately wanted to get the schools and universities on board.

Add a personal development and spiritual element (which I consider to be an extremely valuable addition) and you have a new art which would mould the Japanese youth into better citizens without putting noses out of joint amongst the supporters of the existing Japanese arts. It was a shrewd move. Once I realised this, I was reconciled that I was not adding anything to my karate, I was stripping the inessential away instead.

Chapter 5

A modern Interpretation of Karate ni sente nashi

One of the oldest pieces of legislation in our country (presuming you are reading this in the UK) is that of Common Law. If is from Common Law that we get the fundamental offences like homicide. Common Law also states that a private citizen has a right to defend himself/herself, his/her loved ones and his/her property. This is all good, but there is a grey area attached. The grey area is that the force used must be *reasonable*.

There are other Acts which govern the use of force by law enforcement personnel, such as the Police and Criminal Evidence Act (1984) and they too, mention "reasonable force".

So, what is "reasonable"? Unfortunately, that is usually decided by either a group of prosecutors and defenders, lay persons from a magistrates' bench, or a jury. It will be decided after you have been possibly arrested and interviewed, and you are now standing in the dock in your best suit trying to clarify, in a clinical artificial environment, the feelings and physical symptoms of terror you felt during that violent encounter that occurred at three in the morning in the driving rain on a darkened street six months ago.

The magistrates and the jury are not legal professionals. They are chosen from your peers but, even so, they have to draw their

CHAPTER FIVE

conclusions from witness statements and CCTV footage because they were not there at the time of the incident in question. If any of them have been in your situation, they can probably empathise, but the majority of them will never have been involved in a violent situation and cannot possible know how it feels. (NB: even your Sensei may never have been in a live, violent situation.)

People are all different and the only person who can convey *your* feelings and reactions is you. If the jury find out you are well versed in "martial arts" I guarantee that there will be some amongst them who see those arts through a veil of deadly mystery and will judge you based on that.

This is all very gloomy and I am not saying that should you end up in court you will be damned. I am trying to convey certain realities that you may not have experienced.

Fortunately, some guidance does exist on what can be construed as "reasonable". Basically, it is whatever force is necessary to negate the threat, and no more. Anything above and beyond that is gratuitous violence and would be an aggravating factor in the eyes of the courts. This sounds straightforward enough, but even this can be incident specific.

For instance, if a man attacks you with a baseball bat and you use a walking stick to defend yourself, as long as you stop when the threat is negated, that force can be construed as reasonable. If a man attacks you with his bare hands and you use the same walking stick in the same manner, you would say that that was excessive.

But what if you were a seventy-six year-old woman? Or the man is twice your size? Or he is simply the first person to get to you out of a gang of six who all intend doing you harm? The definition of reasonable force is not as cut and dried as legislation would have us believe. Every situation is different and, if the courts are doing their jobs correctly, all factors should be taken into account before it is decided whether the force used is reasonable.

So what can you do? First of all, there is nothing glamorous

CHAPTER FIVE

about violence, no matter what films would have you believe. If you have any sense at all (and any grasp of the philosophical side of karate) you will avoid violence like the plague. If a violent encounter is unavoidable, stop when the threat is negated.

Should the police become involved, whether you are giving a witness statement or are being interviewed under caution, make sure you go on record explaining exactly how you felt when the incident occurred. There is no room for bravado and ego; if you felt fear, tell them. If there were other factors conditioning your actions, such as the feeling that if he got past you, your family was in danger, mention it. Stressful situations, such as being placed under arrest or being interviewed under caution, can cause time to seemingly fly by and, before you know it, your opportunity to relate your experience of the incident will have passed, so try and keep your wits about you.

You need to hope for the best but plan for the worst. If you are going to find yourself in a court, you need to help the people judging your guilt to understand why you did what you did, to put them, figuratively speaking, in your shoes.

Do not forget though: your comments about the fear you felt and why you did what you did will only be effective if they are true. There will be people other than you speaking to the police and in the courts.

So, when we talk about reasonable force, does that mean we have to wait until we are physically attacked before we can act? The short answer is: No. The law allows what is called a "pre-emptive strike" if you have a *reasonable and honest belief* that you are in danger. What is construed as *reasonable and honest belief* is down to you to prove in the aftermath of the encounter, but would depend on lots of factors which would probably be unique to that situation.

Understanding body language and the imminent physical signs on a human body which imply an intention to fight and that violence is imminent can greatly assist in this.

CHAPTER FIVE

Although this is not true in every encounter, usually, when the fight ritual begins, your opponent will try to make himself seem larger. He will push out his chest and spread his arms. His face will redden, and he may shout. This is designed to make you back down as soon as the situation begins and to "scare" you away.

As I said, every situation is unique and if, for whatever reason, you decide to stay, you will be witness to the next step in the ritual. This is when the body prepares itself for actual conflict. Your opponent's limbs will come back in closer to the body, his face will pale as his speeding heart spreads blood to his organs to cope with the chemical reactions as his body prepares for fight or flight. His chin will instinctively drop and, in complete contrast to the first part of the ritual, he will make himself appear smaller in an instinctive effort to present a smaller target. He may look away from your eyes to a potential target area and his fists may clench.

These symptoms, or variations of them, may or may not appear, but knowing them when they *do* appear can give you that reasonable and honest belief that you are going to be attacked.

It is also surprisingly common for people to make some comment, such as "I'm going to fucking smack you" before attacking. I am at a loss as to why you would advertise your intentions in this manner, but it does occur. If there are any psychology buffs out there who can tell me, I would be most grateful.

So, interesting and necessary as learning all this is, how does it fit in with our continuing quest to make our karate more pragmatic whilst adhering to the original philosophical concepts?

There is a concept in karate known as *karate ni sente nashi,* roughly translated as "there is no first attack in karate". This tends to imply that a *karateka* must wait for their opponent to make the first move before going into action. In traditional karate, this "first attack" has, in my opinion, been somewhat misconstrued.

Taking the concept of *karate ni sente nashi* into our modern scenario, you may think that a pre-emptive strike goes against this

CHAPTER FIVE

concept. I don't think it does. What needs to be established is: *At what point does an attack begin?* This concept has always been taken as though the first attack is a physical one, such as a grab or a strike, but it does not have to be. As soon as you have that reasonable and honest belief, the *second* that feeling of being under immediate threat kicks in, the attack has begun. It may be subtle, such as an invasion of your personal space, the clenching of a fist or a comment, but it is the point where you can put your hand on your heart and say that what you did was justified.

Karate ni sente nashi, therefore, merely means that the *karateka* should never seek out physical confrontation, should never be the protagonist. But should imminent violence become a reality, it must be identified and negated as quickly as possible. This opens the door for the pre-emptive strike to enter your arsenal without veering from the *do*.

Part 2
THE INTERNAL

(mindful self-protection)

Chapter 6

Zanshin and Mushin

Both these words will be familiar to most, if not all, students of any Japanese martial art.

Zanshin is the state of complete awareness that a martial artist must cultivate. He must be in total touch with his environment and any potential threat that exists within it.

Now, I was taught that, when performing *kata*, I should enter a state of *zanshin* for the duration of the *kata* and not "switch it off" until *yamae* was called by the sensei.

Why? Am I only to be aware whilst I am in the middle of a violent situation? Could it be that a lack of said awareness got me into this situation in the first place?

In my opinion, *zanshin* should be cultivated all the time. When you take it to its grass roots level, *zanshin* is the application of common-sense threat awareness.

Mushin is the concept whereby the mind is completely calm and uncluttered at the point of conflict. There is a wonderful scene in the film *The Last Samurai* where Nobutada tries to give Aldgren (played by Tom Cruise) advice about why he lost a friendly challenge match. He tells him he has "too many minds". He "minds" that people are watching, he "minds" his opponent, he "minds" his sword. Nobutada finishes the lecture with the phrase "no mind". This is the essence of *mushin*.

CHAPTER SIX

In real life the mental clutter that precedes violent confrontation can take many forms. You may know your attacker and know he has a reputation for being a good fighter, so your subconscious will start asking if you are up to the challenge. What if you lose? Your friends may be with you, who know you are skilled in some kind of martial art and will no doubt expect some magical effortless victory on your behalf. This puts added pressure on you. You may have your family with you, who may be at risk if your attacker gets past you.

You will also have the mental juggling of what technique you are going to use and be suffering the effects of an adrenalin dump: tunnel vision, auditory exclusion, shaking limbs.

And then, because your mind can be insidiously versatile when it comes to undermining you, it will flip the coin and make you worry about what will happen if you win. What if you are arrested for injuring your attacker? Yes, you can claim the use of reasonable force and your right to self-defence, but that will still have to be sorted out after you have been arrested and may even go as far as a trial. What if the attacker wants to take some form of retribution? It might not be against you, it could be a sneak attack on your family, friends, your home or your property. Are you prepared to spend the next six months living in fear?

All these questions will run rampant across your mind in the seconds prior to a violent conflict.

Now, if it is a blitz attack and you have no prior warning, your instinct will kick in and your body will do what it has been trained to do. The mental clutter described above will manifest itself *after* the fight. Using threat awareness should limit the chance of this happening, but there is always a chance that, no matter how careful you are, you could get caught out.

When I was teaching self-defence to the police, we used to try lots of different ways to apply pressure to the students so that they could test their techniques whilst tired, out of breath, even dizzy on one occasion, but nothing can be done in a sterile environment to

CHAPTER SIX

replicate the emotional state someone feels before a live confrontation.

Some people may disagree with me on that, but think about it, even an MMA fighter in a cage is fighting under a set of rules. If he goes to the ground unconscious, the referee steps in – he doesn't have three or four of his opponents' inebriated friends looking to use his head as a football. If he beats his opponent, he is not going to get his windows smashed, his car damaged or his family threatened.

The feelings of trepidation a fighter feels before he steps into the ring or the octagon or onto the mat are very similar to the feelings you will get before a real confrontation, but there are slight differences, and it is these slight differences which can ultimately be your undoing.

Blitz attacks, if *zanshin* is cultivated effectively, should become a rarity and the cultivation of *zanshin* and *mushin* in tandem, what I choose to call "mindful self protection", is not merely the realm of the experienced *karateka*. This mind set can be developed by anyone.

Before we move deeper into mindful self protection, however, it is time for me to impart an ugly truth which I touched on earlier. Bad things *do* happen. It is a simple (if somewhat bleak) fact of life. What a lot of people do not realise, even if they accept that bad things do happen, and this is the hard fact of it, is that they can happen to anybody, *even you*.

So, if bad things do happen, and they can happen to you, does that mean we should all give up? Should we just curl up in a corner and gaze fearfully out at the world?

No. We live our lives as fully as we can. Every day there are people throughout the media telling you what is and is not good for you. Eat this, don't eat that. Run, don't run, weight train. There are people who are afraid of flying in case they die, so they sneak off to spark a cigarette up or knock back a neat whisky in the airport at seven in the morning to calm their nerves. Yes, smoking and drinking are harmful, but the effects seem to be somewhat distant. The irony that their lifestyle choice is statistically more dangerous than getting on that plane is lost on them.

What we have to do is realise that not smoking and not drinking, eating the right foods and getting regular exercise, whilst enhancing the quality of your life *now*, are not *guaranteed* to lengthen your life. You could be the fittest man on the planet but you could get hit by a bus. There could be some congenital time bomb ticking away inside your body that you are not aware of. The truth of it is though, that stacking the odds in your favour by adopting a healthy lifestyle actually makes you feel mentally stronger, because you are doing something to tip the scales and any bleak thoughts about what *could* happen no longer enter your head because you have given yourself *peace of mind*.

Yes, you say, bad things can and do happen, but I have done everything in my power to stack the odds in my favour, so what happens next is completely out of my hands and there is nothing I can do about it, so why worry?

We do live in a highly impersonal world where the number of victims of violent crime rises every day and there are people all over the world who, right now, as you read this, are either walking into or suffering through some violent encounter. Please do not fall into the egotistical trap of thinking that because you practise a martial art, you are in less danger than someone who does not. Most martial artists leave it at the dojo door. The concept of self protection is relevant to every single facet of your life, ergo, your karate must be too.

For the layperson, what follows is a series of concepts and strategies designed to enable some degree of peace of mind to enter their lives as far as self-protection is concerned. This is also true for the martial artists reading this, but they must also recognise this as an advanced level of karate training, where the physical takes a supporting role, the internal and mental concepts

CHAPTER SIX

move to the forefront and karate really does begin to exert a positive influence on all aspects of your life.

What follows concerns the cultivation of *zanshin* and *mushin*, and how to go about it.

Chapter 7

The ego

Before we get into the nuts and bolts of "target hardening", I want to spend some time speaking about some of the mental clutter which plagues us in modern life. Clutter which we either need to shed or gain control of before we can begin to cultivate our desired mindset. One aspect of this clutter is the ego.

Some of you may be wondering what this has to do with self-protection, but please, bear with me, all will become clear.

Dictionary.com carries this definition of "ego":

1. The "i" or self of any person, a person as thinking, feeling and willing and distinguishing itself from the selves of others and from objects of its thought.
2. Psychoanalytically, the part of the psychic apparatus that experiences and reacts to the outside world and thus mediates between the primitive desires of the Id and the demands of the social and physical environment.
3. Egotism: conceit, self importance.
4. Self esteem or self image: feelings (e.g. "wounding" the ego)
5. Scholasticism: a) the enduring and conscious element that knows experience and b) the complete person comprising both body and soul.

CHAPTER SEVEN

6. Ethno: a person who serves as a constant reference point in the study of organisational and kinship relationships.

This is quite a hefty, seemingly far-reaching definition but, put simply, the "ego" as psychologists understand it arose from man trying to learn how we came to be what we are. What constitutes an "ego" has always been there, obviously, but a seemingly random collection of thoughts and impulses is now given some cohesion and an umbrella under which to shelter.

Some parts of the definition are necessary components of a psyche in order for a person to function effectively within the set boundaries of our culture and modern society. For instance, the psychoanalytical definition at point 2 implies that the ego is in place to act as a form of control mechanism.

The id covers our primal impulses. This is where the need for shelter, food and perpetuating our species comes from. In order for human beings to function effectively these desires must be met, but in a controlled way. When this control mechanism is bypassed we enter the realm of crime and violence.

The above definition would have us believe that acting in a criminal or violent manner is an acquiescence to the id with no thought of society or the impact upon it such deeds may cause. But is it? Are the transgressors giving in to the primal desires or are they operating under the influence of selfishness brought on by a controlling ego?

This is an extremely complex debate, which this definition tends to gloss over, and it very much depends upon the individual driving force for each person.

The desire for sexual reproduction, whilst based in the id and intended to ensure that our species does not become extinct, has now been twisted so that the end result (pregnancy, birth and hence the perpetuation of the species) is carefully controlled, occurring, in most cases, when we wish it to, leaving us free to pursue the pleasurable bit without having to worry about the consequences.

CHAPTER SEVEN

There is nothing wrong with this until the boundaries are crossed. In our society sexual intercourse can only take place with a willing mate. Rape is a vile intrusive act that ruins lives and it cannot be argued in any way that rapists are giving in to their *need* to procreate, because, being honest, sex is no longer about that and hasn't been for some considerable time, and a lot of the time the sex act is merely a weapon for rapists. It is the *power* over their victims that they enjoy. Now, you tell me that is not driven by ego.

This is but one example, but it illustrates my point.

In addition, I have an issue with the first part of the definition too. It is not that it is wrong, it is that it is *right*. It speaks of identifying the self as separate from other persons and other objects. On the face of it, this would seem a harmless viewpoint from which to interact with the world.

In fact, this is the root of one of the main problems in our world today. The separation of the "self" from the rest is merely fuel for the ego. A "protective barrier" is erected between "you" and "everything else", severing a vital connection. This barrier is nothing more than an illusion constructed by your psyche as the ego exerts its control.

On a small scale, generally speaking, we are a social species with an inbuilt need to interact and seek companionship, but we are forced to do so from behind an ego-constructed "shell" which, often subconsciously, we have wrapped around ourselves.

On a larger scale (I was going to use the word "grander" but there is nothing grand about it) we have what we are doing to our planet. Our individual ego lives alongside our "species ego", whereby we see ourselves as the primary species on the planet and some of us (thankfully not all) think we can treat the other species, the flora and fauna and, indeed the planet itself, as we see fit and hang the consequences. This is ultimately self-defeating for our species too; if the planet dies, so do we.

CHAPTER SEVEN

Point 3 of the definition speaks of conceit and self importance. The truth is that everyone *is* important, but no more or less than anyone else, and no more or less than any of the other species of plants and animals around us. The problem arises when the importance one feels about oneself becomes unrealistically elevated, the ego becomes bloated and then we enter the realm of conceit.

If you want to argue that we are the most important species on our planet, just think for a moment about all the things the planet, and life thereon, could not live without. We are not on that list. In fact, if we were being truthful, the world would be better off without us. We are all take and no give. Without the intervention of humans, the atmosphere would not be depleting, the eco-systems of the world would not be suffering deforestation and changing climates and animals would face extinction only through natural selection. If we were to be wiped off the face of the earth tomorrow, the sad truth is that life would go on, and would probably be better for it.

We are here, however, and we have the same in-built survival instinct that the rest of the animal kingdom has. What we need to do is stop lording it over everything else, including each other.

So, "self importance" in this context is not good, whereas realising your worth in the grand scheme of things is good and, no matter who you are, that worth will be there if you look for it.

Chapter 8

"Positive" and "negative" ego

Now that we have looked at how the ego is defined and some of its inherent problems, I want to demonstrate just how deep ego, both individually and collectively, controls and influences our lives.

Healthy Competition?

Can ego be positive? Of course it can. As discussed in the last chapter, it acts as an essential controlling mechanism, but it can also lead us to strive harder to accomplish things.

It remains positive as long as people are aware that there is a balance to be struck. Healthy competition brings out the best in some people and leads to great advances in society. Scientists all over the world want to be the one who finds the cure for cancer, but not just from an altruistic standpoint. Whoever does eventually find it will have secured their place in the history books for eternity (and probably won't have to work ever again). Their research, whilst driven by wanting to eradicate a terrible disease from our society, is also driven by ego, wanting to be "the one". Surely, if this allows us to progress as a species, this kind of ego is good and, from the standpoint of the species, it is. But from the standpoint of an individual, maybe not.

CHAPTER EIGHT

That same ego that drives the successful scientist is also driving the ones who will be ultimately unsuccessful, the ones who are working just as hard but will see nothing for their efforts. How would the failure affect them? Some will accept it graciously and see the good which will arise from their rival's achievement, others will not be able to cope with failure and will self-destruct as a result. This is because the ego does not like to lose.

The Samurai

One section of historical society that fascinates me is the Samurai. Everything they did was governed by Bushido, their code of conduct, which was similar to European Chivalry in that it taught the warrior how to behave, carry himself with dignity and accept death in the correct manner. Accepting the inevitability of death is, I am sure you will agree, essential for any warrior and makes him a formidable opponent on the battlefield. What developed from that, however, was that their acceptance of it mutated into a reverence for a "good" death, which they would actively seek and which, therefore, cheapened their viewpoint on life.

Honour is an essential element to Bushido. Insult the honour of a samurai and he would have your head, especially if you were of a lower caste. In addition, defeat damaged this honour so much that the Samurai could not live with it, and the concept of *seppuku*, or ritual suicide, came into being.

So what is *honour*? If it is dignity and healthy self respect, a reverence for ancestors and older members of society, then that is good. But not being able to stand damage to your *honour* to such an extent that you would take a life (sometimes your own) is the insidious ego exerting its control.

I have read much about the Samurai, especially from the viewpoint of the acceptance of the inevitability of death. Death is something that we don't like to talk about as Westerners, as though if we don't mention it, it might go away. But accepting that it is inevitable is, paradoxically, intensely liberating.

The one aspect I believe branches Bushido down a separate path from chivalry is that of *seppuku*. It speaks of superiors exerting a unhealthy amount of control over their minions and their minion's grim acceptance that this is their lot, instilled in them from birth. It is an ultimately self-defeating action brought about by exertion of, and incorrect acceptance of, the negative ego.

The Search for Faith

Thousands of years ago, deep thinkers pondered our existence and our place in the world. From this arose various religions and belief systems. They arose from nothing more than an attempt to understand the universe around us, how it came to be, and what our place is in it. This understanding is a purely human concept and arises through careful and conscious thought.

No matter what your standpoint, it must be accepted that religion, faith and belief, in their basic pure form (the form they were intended to be) bring comfort and solace to untold millions and have done for millennia. It has set the rules by which many of our societies abide by. We should not steal, we should not kill etc.

The problem with religion/faith/belief is that it requires the interference of humans to survive. Please do not think I am generalising here. There are many people connected to a variety of belief systems who have done nothing but good, the Dalai Lama, Gandhi and Mother Theresa being the most notable examples. What I am referring to is the way humans feel the need to twist faith to their own ends.

People spend millions financing the lifestyles of dubious evangelists in the name of religion and in the hope that their souls will be saved. People have died, and continue to die, simply because they do not believe what others believe. People have been burnt at the stake, gassed in their millions, wiped out by suicide bombers or executed by firing squad simply because their belief system was viewed unfavourably by that of another. This too, is the ego at work.

Politics

People enter the world of politics for a variety of reasons. Politics is there in order that society is run in a just and fair fashion. But how many politicians can say, hand on heart, that that is their sole motivation for entering politics in the first place? Deep down, did they not want to be Prime Minister or President? Was that because they wanted to change the world? Because they wanted to go down in history? To make money? Or all of the above?

I am not saying that pursuing a career for any of these reasons is necessarily a bad thing. As long as the minister understands and accepts his motivations alongside his obligations, then it should all result in something good. As I said at the start of the chapter, ego can be a good thing when it motivates us to advance and excel, but life is all about balance and until we see the ego for what it is, it will always, to some degree, control us when we should be controlling *it*.

Chapter 9

Controlling the ego

I originally intended to call this section *"shedding the ego"*, but the more I thought about it, the more I realised that the ego is not something that can be *shed*. Is it an integral part of every human being. The problem is how much it controls *you* and how much you control *it*.

I once heard somewhere (and I cannot remember where, so if anyone knows its origin please let me know so I can give the source due credit) that comparing yourself to others is ultimately self-defeating. If you perceive they are better than you, your "ego" is bruised because you are not as good as them. If you are better than they are your "ego" becomes inflated, an ultimately fragile pedestal upon which to place yourself as there is always someone better out there and, when you encounter them, your fall will be from a much greater height.

How many great people out there never realised their full potential due to fear of failure? This is your ego holding you back. What after all, is fear of failure? Is it embarrassment because your friends and family would think less of you?

No. It is how you perceive they would react. Any so-called friends who chose to deride you or turn their back on you if you did not succeed were not your friends anyway. True friends would applaud your attempt, successful or not.

CHAPTER NINE

So, if you retain their respect and love whether your endeavours are crowned with success or they crash and burn, why feel fear of failure? It is simply because the ego does not like to lose.

Paradoxically, we have all, at some point in our lives, felt the heat of "peer pressure". If you do not do this, you are a coward. If you do not do this, you cannot possibly hope to be part of our clique. If you do not wear these designer trainers when your friends are all wearing them, you will not fit in. Why? If you are too worried what others will think you will never be able to exert control over your ego.

The truth is - your ego is holding you back through fear of failure, and taking you to a place you do not want to go through peer pressure. The ego does not really know what it wants, apart from an instinct that it does not want to fail.

One of the main concepts in Buddhism is that attachment causes suffering, because ultimately everything changes and whatever you are clinging so desperately to will be lost. This could be a person, a possession, an enjoyable period in your life. It could be anything really. The feeling of clinging and attachment can be construed as coming directly from your ego. It does not like to lose, either conceptually or physically.

So beginning to accept that you are not in control of things as much as you would like and that one day, hard as it may be to accept, things are going to change, will begin to drain strength and power from the self-defeating portion of your ego.

The way you perceive yourself is not the way others see you. The truth is that your own self-importance and your ego place you in a fictitiously elevated position in other people's lives. We need to make an effort to realise that they have their own psyche to contend with. They have problems too, and some may be far more serious than yours.

Try to look at the actions of others in a new light. Is your colleague being sharp with you today because he was born an obnoxious animal? Of course not, he is as much at the mercy of his psyche as you are of yours. The only thing is that you may be able to see that he is actually falling victim to his ego, and so you can be more compassionate when he seems offhand.

Remember though, just because you now know he is the victim of his ego and he does not, it does not make you better than him. Seeing yourself through your position of whether you are better or worse than someone is your ego at work.

Seeing the effects of ego in others does give you a valuable tool. It can stop you from taking things personally. That motorist who remonstrated and gesticulated obscenely at you this morning on your way to work should not make you angry. He does not know you, so how can it be personal? Someone calling you a name is merely sound, vibrations though the air and, although some people can say hurtful things, they are only hurtful from the standpoint of the ego. You do not have to accept that what they say is true, and you don't have to rise to the bait either, that would be relinquishing control over to your ego.

Honest self analysis (keyword: honest) is a wonderful tool. Take a long hard look at yourself. How you treat others, how often you anger, how often you are upset. Think through significant events from your past, particularly ones that make you feel uncomfortable to do so. Some of them may make you squirm with embarrassment, but, as I said, remember that when you recall how badly you dealt with something when you were younger, or you see parts of your past self's personality that you maybe do not like, you are seeing that person through older, more experienced eyes, so do not be too heavy with the judging. What matter is now. The past no longer exists, except in your mind, and even that is not an infallible record.

Now, as you sit thinking about the things you may have done over the years, delve deeper into the ones that cause you concern and ask yourself how many of them could be construed as being motivated by ego. You will find that a surprisingly large number, if not all, are. Analyse it further and try to ascertain the ego's

CHAPTER NINE

motivation. How would you react differently now that you are older and (hopefully) wiser?

The next step is to begin to apply this strategy to the things you do from now on. Sometimes the analysis will have to be quick, while sometimes you will be able to give it a long calculated period of careful thought.

For instance, you are walking home through darkened streets and see a gang of youths on the corner. Now, do you walk straight through the middle of them, risking a pointless confrontation, just to prove to yourself that you are not afraid? Or do you cross the street and carry on your route?

If your honest answer is the former, you are being controlled by your ego. Even if you came out on top, what would you gain? A visit from the police? Reprisal attacks on your home and family?

All you have to do is ignore your ego, and cross the street. How simple is that?

Ask yourself, honestly, whether your actions are motivated by common sense and/or necessity. Almost every action you take can be analysed in this manner. The drive to and from work is necessary and therefore not motivated by ego. Cutting someone up with your car or performing a risky overtake due to impatience during that drive is not motivated by necessity and is your ego attempting to demonstrate that your journey is more important than those of the other motorists.

Are you one of those people who likes a good gossip? Do you hang on every word when someone tells you something juicy about one of your friends or colleagues? This is a very easy trap to fall into (I have been guilty of it myself, I admit). But one of the exercises in controlling your ego is to step outside yourself and views things from the perspective of others. How would it feel if you were the subject of the gossip? (There is every likelihood that you will be, when the others get together without you.) Would it hurt to know that your friends discuss you behind your back? Gossip exists because discussing the failings in others makes you feel better about yourself.

Society, currently, excels in the superficial. Some people are becoming famous through doing not very much at all and the ones who do not become famous model themselves upon the ones that do.

Taking a role model in certain circumstances can be very beneficial. When I was first learning karate I looked at the older more experienced *karateka* around me and, when I saw an aspect of their technique, or their training mindset that I liked, I tried it to see if it worked for me. Sometimes it did, sometimes not, because ultimately, everyone is different. When it *did* work, it obviously made me a better martial artist. The pitfall with role models comes when you no longer want to emulate an aspect of them, you want to be like them *full stop*. An extreme example of this would be the film *Single White Female*, where a room mate does not just model herself on her friend, she tries to become her, with dire consequences.

So by all means have your heroes and role models, but resist the urge to become a sheep and emulate them entirely. This is your negative ego telling you that they are better than you and thus diminishing your sense of self-worth.

When was the last time you opened a newspaper and could not find any scandalous gossip or any bad news about something going on in the world? That is because newspapers are becoming less about reporting the news and more about provoking a reaction. Even if the article is passing on a news item, there will be some criticism hidden within the text to evoke some reaction in the reader. Is this down to the media or the readership?

They would argue that they are printing what people want to read. They are in the business of selling newspapers. If everyone suddenly decided they were no longer interested in scandal and

CHAPTER NINE

gossip in their tabloids, would the media evolve and adapt accordingly?

We, as a race, are subconsciously massaging our group egos by viewing our positions in the world in relation to the positions of others.

Because of modern technology, the world as we see it is a much smaller place. News reaches us from around the globe in the blink of an eye. I talked earlier about the media presenting things to provoke a reaction. Have you noticed that the majority of the news which reaches us from other parts of the globe is usually about some atrocity perpetrated by someone, or a natural disaster?

As I am writing this, people are analysing the capsizing of an Italian cruiser in the Mediterranean which resulted in the loss of many lives. My wife and I discussed a comment that one of the news readers made; she felt the need to tell us that all the British passengers got off safely. Whilst I am obviously pleased that these people survived, does she mean to imply that their lives are more important than the ones from other countries who sadly perished? Or that the ones who died are less important? It could be argued that the comment was probably made to put the minds of their relatives at ease, but by the time she made it, the relatives of those who had died or were still missing had already been informed. It was ill-conceived and illustrates nicely the concept of collective ego and seeing yourself in comparison to others.

I know this section sounds like a diatribe against society in general, but I am merely attempting to illustrate the traps and pitfalls the ego creates whilst you are moving through modern life.

In Buddhism, a part of that belief system states that that we are all connected to one another, we all share the same energy if you will. So, if I hurt you, ultimately I am hurting myself. If I do something to damage the world around me, I am damaging myself. Just think about this concept for a moment. No matter what religion, faith or belief you follow, I am sure you can see the sense in this concept, not just in a spiritual sense, but in a practical sense too.

CHAPTER NINE

Being nasty or aggressive upsets others, but it also causes you stress and will take you into situations that you do not want any part of. It is negative ego all the way. We often do not think about what impact we have on others, but it is even rarer we think about the impact of our actions upon ourselves.

As you can see from the above, if we become mindful of the influence of your ego, we will automatically detach ourselves from a large number of potentially volatile and dangerous situations. If you see the ego for what it is, you will see that it is not as influential, grand or important as it would have you think.

In our day-to-day lives, before we act, we need to think. We need to look at the motivations for our actions. I know a lot of the examples I discussed were nothing to do with self protection, but controlling the ego is not something which you can switch on and off. It must be a constant practice, and it must start small. The control needs to be cultivated through your day-to-day life so that, when you most need it, it will be there instinctively. Learning to control your ego, so that it does not take you into places and situations you do not want to be in, is an important aspect of self-protection with other far-reaching benefits. It will make you a better person too.

Chapter 10

Fear

There is an episode in season 4 of the 20th Century Fox TV series Buffy the Vampire Slayer, starring Sarah Michelle Gellar, which is based entirely around the concept of fear. During a Hallowe'en party, an ancient symbol is accidentally activated and everyone begins to experience their worst fears. This is all apparently caused by a demon which feeds on fear. The demon itself look hideous in the textbook and they are all dreading encountering it. But when it does appear, towards the end of the episode, it is about two inches tall.

This very effectively illustrates how what we perceive as fear can become grossly exaggerated and all consuming, when actually there is very little substance to it at all.

Sometimes our fears arise from past experience. I personally have a problem with small spaces and being in the middle of crowds. This comes from being trapped in the partially-submerged car. I know this because the problem was not apparent before then. Some days it is very intense, other days not so much.

My wife has a phobia of snakes, while my daughter is terrified of spiders. This is despite the fact that we live in a country where the spiders are small and harmless and, although we have snakes, you hardly ever see them in the wild.

Phobias such as these are fear in the strictest sense, as they are borne from a need to survive. My claustrophobia comes from

CHAPTER TEN

almost dying in that accident. My wife and daughter have their phobias because, subconsciously, the mid-brain tells them that the animals they fear can endanger their lives.

Some people are afraid of the dark. On the surface of it we can say that this is because they have an overactive imagination, but taking it to an instinctive level, when we are in complete darkness we are vulnerable. In days gone by, darkness equated to vulnerability from predators and from enemies.

People with a fear of heights feel on an instinctive level that if they fall, they will be hurt or killed. It is a subconscious defence mechanism in the human body. The fear of not surviving is the one true fear we have.

Phobias can, ultimately be worked through and, in some cases eradicated entirely through the use of certain techniques. But people only tend to find help for their phobias if they have an adverse effect upon the rest of their lives, because it takes a lot of work.

If you have an intense fear of heights, would you voluntarily join a climbing club? Of course not, how would that be fun? But if your fear was causing other aspects of your life to suffer, for instance if your company moved to new offices and you had a window looking out of the twentieth floor, you might consider learning to climb in a controlled environment would help you immensely in controlling or even conquering your fear.

The survival instinct is hard wired into our psyche. We could not perpetuate our species effectively without it, and you can see it throughout the animal kingdom. Animals evolve to adapt in the best way to their environment to increase their chances of survival.

Humans, from a psychological standpoint, are extraordinarily complex and our society has created a host of *lesser* fears which can plague us. They range from fear of our homes being broken into and fear of being the victim of a rape or a robbery through to fear of public speaking, even, for martial artists, a fear that their techniques might not work in a live situation. There are a lot of fears

CHAPTER TEN

that are borne out of the ego, such as fear of not fitting in, and fear of failure, which we have already covered.

Now, you may have a fear of public speaking, but be required to give an important presentation, or you may have an interview for a job you really want. You will be excited at first, then as the day of the presentation or interview draws close, the excitement will become anxiety. You will lose sleep and become irritable and uncommunicative because all you can think about is the horrendous experience which awaits you.

On an instinctive level, this fear is borne from the fact that, during the presentation, you will feel exposed standing in front of all those people and will therefore feel vulnerable. During the interview situation, you have acceded power to the interview panel and are at their mercy because you want this job, ergo, you are vulnerable.

Vulnerability equals extinction as far as your survival instinct is concerned so, even though, in the grand scheme of things, the presentation and job interview are not a direct threat to your survival, your subconscious equates that vulnerability to a survival situation and the chemical reactions inside your body giving rise to your fear are no different from those which would happen internally if you were attacked.

The survival instinct has not evolved as the rest of our bodies, and the world around us, have. It is an instinct. It is not borne of rational thought, it is the Id, and it is a part of every animal on the planet on an elemental level. Psychologists call it the *fight or flight response* because it comes from a need to survive, so the body prepares itself to either fight or run. Heart rate increases to drive blood to various parts of the body you will need to rely on. You will have an intense desire to visit the toilet, because your body wants to dump excess weight (this is the reason people have been known to lose control of their bladders in terrifying situations). In the extreme the adrenalin will give you tunnel vision, because you only need to see either your enemy or your escape route.

CHAPTER TEN

You may also suffer something called auditory exclusion, where your hearing appears to partially shut down. This comes from the fact that you do not need to hear to fight or run away. These, and a host of other minor chemical reactions will fire off in your body when the fight or flight response kicks in.

There is a caveat to the fight or flight response though. It is meant to be a short term experience, designed to last just long enough to get you out of danger. Whether that is to give you a turn of speed to run away, or an enhanced burst of strength and speed to fight, it is not meant to be sustained for a long period of time. The chemical reactions in your body, and the effect of the fight-or-flight response, can have a damaging effect if sustained over a long period. They can lead to heart and blood pressure problems, to name but two.

So, what we now call "stress" is actually symptoms from our survival instinct in our mid brain manifesting themselves when they are not really needed. Recognising these symptoms within your own body and seeing them for what they are can alleviate them to a great degree.

In addition, one thing which happens when you get these reactions in your body is that your breathing pattern changes. Your breathing becomes fast and shallow as you try to get as much oxygen into your system as possible ready for the action phase. Now in the short term this is fine, but over a sustained period of time this can be extremely harmful.

The easiest way to alleviate the symptoms of fight or flight is through *correct* breathing. Read any book about *yoga* or *qi gong* and it will mention the importance of correct breathing. As we grow into adulthood, the way we breathe changes. When we are babies, we use our entire lungs, so that when we breathe in, the abdomen expands rather than the chest, and when we breathe out, the abdomen contracts. Adults tend to breathe in the upper portion of their chest, which makes their breath shallow and does not using the entire respiratory mechanism to its fullest potential.

CHAPTER TEN

Find somewhere quiet and just sit for a moment. Keep your body relaxed and your back straight. Close your eyes if it helps. Now, inhale deeply through your nose, hold it for a few seconds, then exhale slowly and thoroughly through your mouth, feeling as if you are emptying your body completely.

What was your body's reaction to the breath? If your shoulders hunched and your chest expanded, the breathing was shallow and taking place in your upper body. The sensation you are seeking is for your shoulders to remain down and relaxed and the abdomen to flex outwards as you inhale and then to flatten as you exhale. When you first try it, it may be a struggle and feel somewhat artificial, as beginners tend to flex their abdomen outwards to an unnecessary degree. Eventually though, with sustained practice, your body will *remember* and your breathing will become instinctive and deep once more, the way it should be.

Controlling your breathing can go a long way to alleviating fear. Through being mindful of your breath you may find that you do not suffer stress as readily as you used to. Taking a few deep, slow, correct breaths tells your body that you are calm, and that there is no threat to your wellbeing. Like a chain reaction, this is subconsciously felt throughout the body and the symptoms of fight or flight simply fade away.

As well as controlling your breathing, look at the fears you currently suffer from. Do not just say, "I'm afraid of X", and leave it at that. Think about where the fear originates. Are you afraid of X because it is a direct threat to your survival? If it is not, then what your body is interpreting as fear must be due to some aspect of it triggering the primitive survival instinct. If you can think it through, you may find the part of your fear that is actually causing the reaction and hence be able to combat it. For instance, do not leave it at the level of "I don't like spiders because they are disgusting, they are hairy and have too many legs." Those are ground for disliking the appearance of something, not being afraid of it. Go deeper than that.

CHAPTER TEN

Let's just return to the job interview for a moment. I am sure you have heard the old technique for combatting interview nerves whereby you picture the interview panel in their underwear. Have you ever given some thought as to why this works?

On the face of it, imagining these people in their underwear can be very amusing and your psyche knows that amusing situations are not a threat to your survival, so your stress level tends to decrease, but it is also the transference of vulnerability.

As I stated earlier, you are submitting the control of your life and destiny over to these people who may, or may not, give you the job of your dreams. This makes you feel the vulnerability which causes the survival instinct to kick in. In situations such as the technique discussed here, the vulnerability is transferred to the interview panel and diminishes their perceived power over you. This tells your instincts that you are no longer vulnerable and calms your nerves.

So, take it to an instinctive level. Ask yourself if this fear is a direct threat to your survival. It will put your fears in perspective and may be extremely empowering for you too.

Of course, many of our fears are of things which are less substantial, sometimes things which have not happened yet, and might never occur. We will look at these next.

Chapter 11

Future "Fears"

In Gavin de Becker's excellent book *The Gift of Fear* (see bibliography), he talks at some length about these kinds of fear. He states that fear that something *might* happen, for instance the fear that someone might break into your house, cannot really be classified as a fear *per se*, as it is not an immediate threat.

In the last chapter we spoke about the inbuilt survival instinct and the chemical reactions it causes in the body. Remember it is only supposed to be a short-term solution. Can you imagine the harm you could cause yourself if such a fear caused those reactions to be there more or less constantly, on a slow trickle as it were?

The fear of some future event which may not even happen is a purely human concept. We are able to rationalise and organise our lives, so we can take measures to lessen the likelihood of such things occurring, but because something still *might* happen, that feeling can always be there.

De Becker talks about worry and anxiety being purely human concepts, and he is absolutely right. The rest of the animal kingdom operates on a far more primal level. The need for food, procreation and shelter, the Id side of things, pretty much dominates their lives. Because we are intelligent, and have built such a vast interactive society, many of the things wild animals need and have to hunt for are handed to us on a platter. (I realise I am generalising and that

CHAPTER ELEVEN

there are parts of the world where human beings, merely through being born in a certain place, are denied the things that many of us take for granted, but I am merely using these examples to illustrate my point).

Supermarkets and malls place all our needs for food and comfort in one handy place. We build up cities, conurbations and vast areas of urban sprawl so we can live alongside other humans and interact. For people in most societies, it is made very easy to bring a child into the world and feed and clothe it.

So if our base needs are handed to us on a platter, what does our mind dwell on? The problem with a highly-developed frontal lobe giving us the ability for deep and rational thought is that when the thoughts are not dwelling on our immediate survival, they run off on their own.

At the risk of going deep and philosophical for a moment, what exactly *are* your thoughts? And how do you know they are yours? There is a lot of text out there, particularly from the Buddhist angle, about what the mind actually is.

When you go to sleep, your body shuts down to recharge, so to speak, but the mind does not. It carries on working, creating dreams in your subconscious as it sorts everything into place that you have thought of or encountered that day.

Sometimes it plays on fears that you may not even know you have and gives you a nightmare. Bram Stoker wrote *Dracula* after having a nightmare brought on by eating dressed crab. As least, that's what he put it down to. Have you ever heard the tale that eating cheese just before bed will cause you to have nightmares? It is probably due to the fact that some rich foods are hard to digest and make your body work hard when it is supposed to be shutting down for a while. This confusion manifests itself in your mind, hence the nightmares.

So, on the face of it, your mind and your thoughts are very much a part of you. But are they? Think back to an event from your past.

CHAPTER ELEVEN

Whether it is a good memory or a bad one does not matter, but it must not be recent and it must be something which happened directly to you, not something you watched someone else do.

Really concentrate. Close your eyes and immerse yourself deeply into the memory. Now, are you seeing the event through your own eyes as though you are reliving the experience? Or are you seeing things from the perception of a fictitious third person? Nine times out of ten it will be a mixture of both. So who is this third person whose perception you have? It could be that it is your mind filling in gaps in your memory by recalling photos or film recordings from the event and giving you that view, but I do not think so.

When I think back to being stuck in that car, my mind flits from first to third person, and there are no photos or film footage of that. When I think about the grading I had for my *shodan*, way back in 1985, I see it from both "viewpoints" and again, no visual record exists.

Once you have thought about this for a while, try another experiment. Think about the event again, and then ask the question, "Who is thinking these thoughts?" If you can step outside what you perceive as your mind, we are back to the question - are the thoughts really *yours?*

These are the same thoughts that give you the worry and anxiety about some future negative event that may or may not happen, and they might not even be yours. The problem with these kinds of thoughts is that they are self sustaining. Say you feel anxiety because next Wednesday you have a long car journey to make and are fearful of an accident. Once you complete that journey, that particular anxiety is no more, but the negative thoughts will merely shift onto something else, and the process starts again. Have you ever heard of someone described as a born worrier? This is the cycle that they find themselves trapped in.

In order for the cycle to be broken, it is essential for the sufferer to recognise the "fears" for what they are. The thoughts need to be

CHAPTER ELEVEN

reined in, so to speak, and the mind not allowed to *wander*. This is a perfect description of what the mind actually does.

If you kept a horse as a pet, you would keep it tethered, or safely ensconced in a stable. If you did not, it would wander off on its own. This is exactly like your mind. It might belong to you, but unless you keep it tethered, it will wander off and get itself into trouble.

Like most things which are worth doing, this I not easy, and for a time at least it requires constant vigilance in your thoughts. Whenever anxious or negative thoughts arise, it might help if you think "These thoughts are not mine anyway". This distances you somewhat from the negative thoughts and goes some way to severing your connection to them. This is yet another aspect of attachment causing suffering. If you attach yourself to your thoughts and identify with them too deeply, suffering ensues.

As I said at the very start of this section, bad things can and do happen, but if you have done everything you can as an individual to minimise that risk, whatever happens next would be completely out of your hands.

Remember the old Buddhist saying:

"If something is troubling you and you can sort it out, sort it out and stop worrying. If something is troubling you and you cannot sort it out, accept that it is beyond your control and stop worrying."

I also saw a good one on a plaque one of my colleagues used to have on her desk:

"Lord, grant me the serenity to accept the things I cannot change, the courage to change the things I cannot accept, and the wisdom to know the difference."

If you are a born worrier, it will take time to change something that is so deeply ingrained into your psyche. Start small. Think about

CHAPTER ELEVEN

something that makes you anxious. Is it an outcome over which you have some degree of control? If the answer is yes, do what is necessary and defeat the negative thoughts from within. If the answer is no, train yourself to step outside these thoughts and defeat them by distancing yourself from them and recognising them for what they are.

One way to stop anxiety about future events, and stop letting past events control your present and future fears, is the concept that lies at the crux of *zanshin, mushin* and Mindful Self Protection. So that is where we are going next.

Chapter 12

Now is all there is

I was going to name this chapter "What is now?" but it sounded like a Zen koan. The truth is that "now" is all there is.

There is only the present moment and even as you begin to think about this, that moment is gone. We have labelled the movement from moment to moment as the concept of *time*, but this is a purely human invention. Animals and plants have no concept of the passage of time; even the sentient ones follow their instincts far more than we do.

The problem with the concept of time is that, much like our ego, we are very much controlled by it. Sometimes, obviously this is necessary. There is no point calling a meeting for instance, or arranging a karate class, if you do not specify a time. These are occasions when groups of people need to come together at one time in one place for the meeting/class to function effectively. Without the addition of a set time we only have confusion.

Time is also essential for the study of history, especially when it comes to things like carbon dating and assessing when discoveries were made. Without some concept of dates and times, historical studies could not take place.

Time only becomes a problem for us when we are made too aware of the passage of it. Deadlines are set at work which must be met (I have a good friend who is a PA and often has tenders

CHAPTER TWELVE

which have to be submitted to a deadline, which causes her no end of stress until they are in and consumes both her working life and home life), our working days are governed by having to be at certain places at certain times. We become so focused in that future date or time that we lose sight of the moments we are in now.

Have you ever noticed though, that when you are waiting for something you are looking forward to, time seems to pass much more slowly? Your favourite band is coming to a city near you in three months time. You already have the tickets, but it seems like ages until the time finally arrives. For children, as I dimly recall, Christmas Eve must qualify as the longest day of the year. Time seems to move more slowly in these instances, because we become acutely aware of each passing moment, counting it down gradually, instead of becoming so immersed in our lives that time flies.

Ideally, we need to capture that feeling (not the frustration that the desired event is a long time coming, but the awareness of each passing moment), harness it, and put it to use throughout the rest of our lives too. Imagine that feeling that time is moving so slowly, but put a positive spin on it. You are actually alive to each moment and, all of a sudden, you seem to have ample time to accomplish your goals because you are using your time more efficiently.

We wake when our alarm clocks force us to. Some, like myself, get up before the rest of the people in the house and are gone before the others get up, driving to work through cold, dark, quiet streets on autopilot in order to get to work on time. My wife has to factor in getting our daughter ready for school and has the timing down to a fine art, getting breakfast for them both and getting them both dressed and ready to go seconds before they need to get in the car.

Children are dropped off at school at appointed times, shifts start at work, and the day is made up by a series of mini deadlines that have to be met. When the shift ends, everything happens in reverse. The children are picked up from school, taken home and

CHAPTER TWELVE

badgered into doing their homework until everyone sits down to tea and then the pots are washed, the children are bathed and put to bed and the parents collapse into their armchairs exhausted, grabbing a little alone time before going to bed and getting a few hours' sleep, ready to do it all again.

Our entire lives are governed by looking at the clock and being all too aware that we must be at certain places at certain times. For some, hobbies and pastimes provide a welcome distraction, but even these must be fitted in around the more important aspects of our lives.

Now, being mindful and being in the present moment does not mean that any of this will change, or that responsibilities will be neglected. It simply means that you become totally immersed in the given moment and give it your fullest attention possible.

We spend an inordinate amount of time thinking about what we have yet to do, even at the expense of thinking about what we are doing right now. People hustle and bustle through their day, harassed because they have so much left to do and so little time to do it in.

The truth is (and this is so unbelievably simple) you can only do one thing at once. Multi-tasking is a myth. It's like those magicians who spin plates on top of those thin flexible poles or people who juggle with several objects at once. It is actually merely a very fast sequence of single tasks.

Take the juggler for instance. He catches the knife whilst the orange is still in the air and then throws the knife aloft before catching the ball. His brain does not do all these things at once. While the knife is being caught and thrown, it is all his mind is focusing on. Once it has been thrown with the correct weight and trajectory, he is then free to forget about it (even if he does not realise it) because the laws of physics tell him what will happen to it while he turns his thoughts to the orange, which is falling towards his hand once more. This then becomes the focus until the orange is correctly airborne again, and so it goes on.

CHAPTER TWELVE

A busy housewife will have the washing and vacuuming to do, but it is physically impossible to do both at the same time. She will put the first load in the washing machine and then vacuum the living room and dining room whilst that cycle is complete. She will then move away from the vacuum cleaner, back to the washing to swap that load to the dryer or the washing line, then put another load in before she returns to vacuuming the bedrooms.

What we perceive as multi-tasking is actually the completion of small incremental steps leading us, in stages, to an accomplished task, which we do alongside other incremental steps for a separate task. Although the main tasks appear to be completed at the same time, we are actually just doing small portions of each project. We keep going in this manner until all the jobs are complete.

The one concession I will give, the one thing that comes close to multi-tasking, is doing your daily chores whilst in the role of parent. But even this is not technically multi-tasking. Being aware of your child, and mindful of their safety, is merely an extension of being mindful for your own safety. More on this later.

The reason we get so stressed in these situations is because our mind dwells upon what remains to be done, even though we are working diligently to accomplish all our set goals. This is especially true when our tasks are routine and mundane. Granted, it does not take much thought to heave a pile of clothes out of a washer and into the dryer, so the mind thinks about other things. When we are busy, these "other things" are inevitably the other things we need to complete. But what if, as you are removing the damp clothes from the washing machine, you breathe deeply and take in the scent of the fabric softener? What if, as you walk outside, you take a second to bask in the sunlight and, as you put the clothes on the line, you become acutely aware of the different textures and fabrics running through your hands?

I know this sounds fluffy, deep and spiritual, but if you were fully immersed in your task and giving it your full attention, these are the kinds of things you would notice.

CHAPTER TWELVE

The concept of living fully in each moment means that the past and present do not actually exist. Even our memories and recollections become distorted over time, so that what we perceive about the past is not a true record. It is based on the way we felt at the time and the way we feel now. It is also extremely selective and buries the more unpleasant memories to protect us. I spent my teenage years in the eighties, my parents spent theirs in the sixties. Ask anyone from any generation and they will say that theirs was the best time to be alive. This is pure nostalgia. During the eighties we had soaring unemployment, riots, the Hillsborough disaster, the Bradford fire, the miners' strike, the Falklands War, the unrest in Northern Ireland spilling over onto the mainland, the advent of AIDS, massive famine in Africa and the Lockerbie bombing. So, how can my recollection that the eighties were a fantastic time to be alive be true? For millions of people it was hell on earth. My recollection is not your recollection, so how can the past be seen to exist with any consistency?

I can remember a quote in an old Shaun Hutson book, (I think it was *White Ghost)* where the main character, Shaun Doyle, is calling the members of the French Resistance terrorists. His supervising officer argues they were not terrorists and Doyle, quite rightly, counters "They were if you were German", which is perfectly true and illustrates the different ways the past can be perceived.

We can state, with fair certainty, that the sun will come up tomorrow, and that time will continue to pass at the same rate (although as you get older it seems to go faster) but this is not based on future prediction, it is based upon experience.

This is the one aspect of the past that has a bearing on the present but is more to do with generalities than with details. In autumn, the winter fashions will arrive in the shops because we can be fairly sure it is going to get colder as the year progresses. We are not predicting the future, we are merely basing it on what our experience of the world around us has put us through before.

CHAPTER TWELVE

The future is unwritten and until it happens (when it becomes the present anyway) it is nothing but a concept. We have no way of knowing what is around the corner. Worrying about the future is fruitless because we have no idea what it holds.

I had a bit of a discussion with a colleague about this concept once and he mentioned shopping lists. I intend to talk in depth about lists later on but, basically, he was saying that writing a shopping list meant that you were concentrating more on the future than the present moment. Did it? In the present moment you are thinking about what you need from the shops and are planning for the inevitable fact that you and your family need to eat over the coming week. You are merely making a list. The fact that the list pertains to future meals does not matter. The present moment, therefore, is the preparation of the list, not the shopping or the eating of the food.

Immersing yourself in the present moment also ties in with the section on ego and the section on fear. Striving to feed the ego is often based upon past glories, or past events which push us into situations we should rightly be avoiding. Immersion in the present moment means that the past events have no power over us because they do not actually exist.

The fear aspect comes back again to the survival risk. Any threat to our survival is instantaneous and must be dealt with there and then. Anything else falls under the worry or anxiety category and is based on some future event which may or may not happen. The future does not exist, therefore, our worries and anxieties are a waste of energy.

When was the last time you stopped just to look at the sunrise, or the full moon? When was the last time you were aware of every single time you chewed your food and the flavours you were consuming? Did you chew the morsel until it had no more flavour to give? If you were fully in the present moment you would do just that. Too many of us rush through our lives with our heads down, letting

CHAPTER TWELVE

a myriad wonderful things pass us by and go unnoticed because our minds are elsewhere.

Leaving aside the obvious benefits on stress levels and spirituality and the general feeling of wellbeing that living in the moment provides, there is another factor to consider. Living in the present moment will drastically reduce your chances of being singled out as a victim.

Chapter 13

The perils of preoccupation

"He just came out of nowhere"
"The attack was totally unprovoked"
"I never got a good look at him"

I have heard these comments, or at least variations of them, over and over throughout my career. The people who made the comments were victims of violent crime, sometimes an assault, sometimes a robbery. These are awful, harrowing experiences for anyone, made all the more upsetting and distressing because they can tell us very little about their attacker.

Now, let's look at each one of those comments in turn. Remember, nothing can stop someone trying to do something if they are really determined, but we can try and stack the odds in our favour.

"He just came out of nowhere"

To the unlucky victim of the crime, this is exactly how it looked and felt, but the sad truth is, that most likely, their attacker did not come out of nowhere. Those who engage in violent crime, and in this example we are talking about the opportunist street robber/sexual offender who does not know their victim, do not pick someone at random (even if they think they do).

CHAPTER THIRTEEN

It is the simple and unassailable law of the jungle that is employed by base scavengers and predators in the wild to great effect. The lionesses wander around the herd of wildebeest picking out the weak members, and that is exactly what the criminals do.

Anyone who does not look like "easy pickings" is subconsciously dismissed, and the thought process will usually take milliseconds. A lone offender (which very rarely happens unless it involves an attack on someone far more helpless than they, such as the elderly) will be very selective. Those who hunt in packs may go for riskier prey, depending upon their skill level and bravado.

It must be stressed, these people are not looking for a fight. They are looking to accomplish their goal with a minimum of fuss. For some, it will be money for their next fix, for others it will be some stolen sexual gratification, but all will experience a sick thrill, a buzz, that will likely get them out doing it again and again. The problem with the buzz is that its effects are diminished quickly and greater risks have to be taken to get the same "high". If the offender is carrying out the robbery as a means to an end, for instance for the cash to buy a bag of crack, the buzz means nothing compared to the obtaining of a fix. For those after "street cred" who do it for the thrill, the higher the buzz the better.

Never underestimate a potential offender, because you have no way of knowing which category they belong to until the attack actually starts. What they do not want to do is hang around. The longer they are there, committing their offence, the greater their chances of capture.

A person in their area who walks with their head down, looks preoccupied and harassed, or afraid, is ripe for becoming a victim. They are unaware of their surroundings because their head is down, their mind is on other things and, if they are exhibiting the outward signs of fear, they will be easier to exert control over. Although your physical appearance does play a significant part (I am not being sexist here, I am talking about size and stature) these other factors could be the deciding vote as to whether you get caught out or not.

CHAPTER THIRTEEN

Imagine then, a man or woman who walks tall and is aware of everything going on around them. They see the group on the corner up ahead, they get a good look without being obvious and, whilst not paranoid, they are not complacent either. Without their realising it, these very characteristics will send signals out to the group. I am going to talk about actual target hardening in detail later, but this general level of awareness will remove the feeling that the offender came out of nowhere.

"The attack was totally unprovoked"

This is a difficult one to discuss with victims because the point must be made that, from their point of view, and by their standards, they correctly surmise that they did nothing to provoke what happened to them. This comment, predominantly, was made to me by victims of violent crime after a social night out in a pub or nightclub. The problem was, the low-life who attacked them had a lower set of standards than his victim, a shorter temper and a more tenuous grasp on what constitutes provocation.

Believe it or not, people still venture forth, in this day and age, who do not feel they've had a good night until they have bounced some poor soul off the cobbles. These are often not the people you would expect. Professional people become football hooligans through an attraction to the tribal culture and the adrenalin rush of violent confrontation. The most mild-mannered father/mother/sister/brother/daughter/son can become a beast when under the influence of intoxicants, be they drink or drugs.

The problem is that the victim is often at least as intoxicated as their new enemy and that impairs their judgement and lowers their defences. I am not advocating that you should go teetotal (that, on my part, would be pure hypocrisy) but for some, becoming *too* drunk singles you out as one of the "weak members of the herd" and hence elevates you to the top of their hit list. Another problem with intoxication is that it has an adverse effect on your vision. If you cannot focus very well you look as if you are staring, even if you are not. Staring is a no-no, as some will see it as an outright challenge.

Sadly, there is little I can say that would assist in target hardening if you are intent on venturing into a town centre for an evening out. All I can say is, stay together, don't go too far with the drink (I know, I know, easier said than done) and pick your pubs. Chances are, if you enter an establishment and even the cue ball on the pool table stops rolling to turn and stare at you, you would be best making your excuses and leaving. Leave your ego at home with your car keys.

It is genuinely frightening how vulnerable some people make themselves through intoxication and the use of recreational drugs. The general rule is *know your limits.* If you do, and you exceed them, you have no-one to blame but yourself. Do not fall into the "It'll never happen to me, I'm a martial artist" trap. It can, and chances are, if you push your luck, it will.

"I never got a good look at him."

In some circumstances, this can be deemed an extension of the first comment. If you are so preoccupied that you do not see your attacker until the last minute, chances are you will only remember very little.

Adrenalin is a funny thing. It can make you faster or stronger for fight or flight, but lowers your level of awareness. Auditory exclusion means that you cannot hear as well as you should, tunnel vision limits your field of view and, if the attacker really takes you by surprise, the effects of the adrenalin will last until the attacker is long gone. It is not uncommon for some victims to have gaping holes in their recollections that sometimes do not come back for days (if ever).

CHAPTER THIRTEEN

Your memory will also try and protect you by burying certain aspects of your ordeal. This will render much of what you actually saw unobtainable. Sometimes these can be accessed by a good interviewer (see below), sometimes they are buried a little too deep.

If you were aware of your attacker *before* he or she approached you and you got a good look at them, chances are the aftermath of the adrenalin dump will not hinder that recollection, as the memory was lodged before your body was under duress.

Of course, the ideal would be that you can avoid the attack in the first place, and I am going to try and help you with that a little later.

Another thing to consider is the effect heightened awareness would have on your value as a witness. I know some people out there would rather drink battery acid than put pen to paper on a witness statement, but what if your friend or relative was the victim? Would your views change?

Of course, from the evidential point of view, investigators now have other means at their disposal. They have CCTV and forensic science, which is advancing all the time, so the need for our witnesses to be on the money all the time every time is not as vital as once it was. On the other side of the coin, TV programmes such as the *CSI* series has people believing that forensic science is more than it is and can accomplish things which are seemingly magical. *CSI* is fiction, and a great amount of the equipment and what they do with it is too.

But we also have cognitive interviewing. This is a technique which, in the hands of a trained professional, is an absolute goldmine of a tool. It involves taking the witness back to the situation under scrutiny, mentally placing them back there and recalling all the sensations they experienced at the time.

Too often, we rely solely on our sight when it comes to recalling things, but it is a well-established fact that the olfactory sense triggers more recall and distant memories that recognition by sight does. So our witness suddenly recalls hearing an accent, smelling

CHAPTER THIRTEEN

something unusual or feeling something unusual. This can greatly assist in identifying offenders or locations.

The reliance on sight alone can cause unintentional obstacles too. I recall dealing with a burglary once and a witness, who did not know the offender, saw him fleeing the scene. All they could remember was his hair colour, and the fact that the offender had a tattoo on his neck (although they could not remember what the design was). A suspect was duly located and, inevitably, he denied the offence. This was under the advice of his legal representative, who knew the matter would then progress to an identification parade and, if the witness failed to pick him out, it would seriously undermine the prosecution case.

I was quietly confident that the witness would manage it, and they did, but such is the imbalance in our justice system that one of the identifying marks, the tattoo, was rendered useless because under the rules governing the conduct of ID parades, an artist had to be called in to draw identical tattoos on the other members of the parade (I kid you not). What if the tattoo had been the only thing that the witness could recall? In all likelihood, the burglar would have slipped through the net.

From the point of view of a witness, can you imagine how effective they would be if they were totally immersed in the moment? Do not forget, just because I mentioned that you would appreciate a sunrise, or sniff your washing (so to speak) does not mean that you would wander around in a daze at how magical everything is. It means you would be totally aware of *everything* going on around you. *Zanshin* and *mushin*.

From an investigator's point of view, this would be a dream come true. A witness who could recall absolutely everything, or as good as, does not happen, because we are all lost in our own problems and our own worries/anxieties. This means we do not become aware of situations developing in front of us until they are in full swing.

CHAPTER THIRTEEN

So, we have discussed the perils and pitfalls of being controlled by your ego, and we have discussed the value of living in the moment. Now, I am aware that some people are not interested in mindfulness (the correct term for living in the present moment) from a spiritual point of view and there are plenty of good books out there to tell you how to go about that, but the fact that you are reading this (and haven't cast it aside yet) means that you have at least a passing interest in self-protection and taking your karate beyond the dojo. What I offer next are some practical ways to free your mind to concentrate it on the now, cultivate your level of awareness and make yourself a hard target for any would be attackers.

Part 3
EXTERNAL TECHNIQUES FOR DEVELOPING THE INTERNAL

Chapter 14

The list

My wife tends to poke fun at me from time to time, as I am obsessed with making lists. This is not an OCD (I don't think), however, there is a good reason for it. Making a list of things I have to do over a set period of time frees up my mind to think of other things and stops preoccupation. This may be a list I have compiled for when I get to work, a list of things I have to do at home, or a shopping list.

The difference between my approach and that of my wife, who, as I've already said, is extremely organised, is that I take my list *out* of my head. She will sit on an evening, and tell me everything that she needs to do either the next day or over the coming week. She does not do it to annoy me (so she says), she does it to get things straight in her own mind as to what she needs to do. This means that the coming chores are rolling around loose in her mind and, every so often, she has to gather them up and slip them into some kind of order to reassure herself that she still remembers everything. She then lets them loose again. They stay together for a short while, but it is not long until they are off and running again.

If you have a good memory, or are going through a relatively quiet spell in your life, this mental recollection would be a reasonably easy thing to do. But as soon as you hit a stressful or busy period, your mind will have to return to the mental list more

CHAPTER FOURTEEN

and more often to reassure you that something is not slipping through the cracks.

It is usually, at this point, that my wife concedes defeat and writes things down. She is, paradoxically, incredibly stringent about making a shopping list and this is because she hates shopping and only wants to visit our supermarket once during the week if she can manage it.

So, how will making lists of things to do help you from a self-protection point of view? Simple - it will free a section of your mind that normally holds and collates all the details of the things you need to do, thereby making it easier to root yourself in the present moment.

Even if you do not think the details are there, they are. They are swimming around in your subconscious and they will pop up from time to time to let you know they are still there. This is one of the things that lead to preoccupation and increase your vulnerability when you are out and about. Remember, the people who prey on the vulnerable have 'preoccupation' on their checklist of victim traits, even if they do not realise it. Someone who is distracted will get them salivating like one of Pavlov's dogs hearing the bell.

Now, one of the things that must be in place for the list system to be effective has to be the right mental approach to it. There is no point writing a list and then still running through the things in your mind. As you write or type your list, you must do so *mindfully*. The way to do it is to visualise the list in your mind before you even start to compile a live copy. You must visualise it down to the last detail, the paper, the ink and the actual words you are going to write. If you are typing it onto a device, it actually helps if the imaginary list is in the same font and colour as the text you are typing it in, but more on virtual lists in a little while.

Then, with that list held in your mind, you begin to recreate it on whatever medium you have chosen. As you type the list, use bullet points, and be as brief as possible. Even single words can trigger

CHAPTER FOURTEEN

the memory so that you can remember fully what you need to do. For instance, typing or writing the words "Dry cleaners" on your list is sufficient, rather than, "Take suit to dry cleaners". Sometime, single words are not enough obviously, if you have a list of people you need to contact, the subject matter under discussion should be included to avoid confusion and jog your memory.

Now, as each bullet point is completed on the page, *erase* it from the list in your mind. This might be done with an imaginary eraser, correction fluid, or by mentally highlighting it and pressing delete. I know it sounds weird, but it does work if you give it a chance. Unless you tell your mind to disregard the items, they will stay in your head.

Of course, it is no good making all these lists if you do not put them somewhere you will find them. (If you are actually considering making a list of your lists then your problem is far worse than mine and I urge you to seek professional help.) The beauty of the list system is that you can leave them anywhere. The trick is to leave the list where you will go without having to think.

For instance, a list of the day's chores on the door of the fridge will be there when you go for the milk for your coffee. Work lists should stay at work. At the close of each day, making a list of the things you need to do tomorrow will free up your mind and leave your tasks at work, where they belong. The list can then be stuck on your monitor screen, or in the next page of your diary. Work-related things that *can* be left at work, *should* be. I appreciate that there are times when work intrudes on our home lives, but preoccupation about things you need to do tomorrow and can do nothing about now is a waste of time you could be spending with family and friends.

Personally, I prefer hard copies of my lists where possible. Leaving aside the fact that I am slightly technophobic, electronic devices can, and do, fail, and we do rely on them far too much. If the thought of your phone, or any other data retention device for

CHAPTER FOURTEEN

that matter, dying on you fills you with dread, make sure you have back-ups and pull that worry from your mind. I actually do use the diary on my Android, but it is usually for things I will get reminded about by other means and from other quarters. It comes in handy when I'm arranging other appointments or meetings and need to ascertain my free days, but I do not really need it to remind me of things.

All you fortunate people who have a PA or a secretariat to turn to - do not rely on them too much. I know you employed them for just this kind of thing, but show them some compassion, take some of the pressure off them, and make your own list of your appointments too, just as a back up to theirs. I certainly would not want it on my conscience that my secretary of PA had suffered an attack due to being preoccupied about *my* "to do" list.

It may be that you still find yourself running through the list in your mind at some point. This is the crux of the list-making system. You are making the lists so that you do not have to think about them until it is absolutely necessary to do so. It is all about using your mind correctly, as the tool it is supposed to be. Is it really necessary to be thinking about what you need to do tomorrow whilst you are helping your child with their homework, cuddling up to your partner in front of a DVD or getting to sleep at night? No it is not, and most people would make an effort to blank the things from their mind at this point. Equally important, so you can actually get home to do those things, do you want to be preoccupied with tomorrow's tasks as you are walking towards your car through a darkened car park, or getting the last bus/train home? I wouldn't, and I don't think you would either.

Chapter 15

The commentary

Now that you are no longer moving through life preoccupied by all the things you need to do, your mind is free to begin to pay proper attention to the world around you. Granted, there are always going to be worries and anxieties that will creep into your mind. Concerns about the health of a loved one, for instance can be a strong and justifiable distraction.

Earlier in the text we have talked about fears, worries and anxieties and the need to keep them in control, but, even with the best of intentions, we can sometimes "fall off the wagon".

What you need now is something to occupy your mind when you leave the sanctity of your home that will keep you focused upon your safety and will also mean that your worries and anxieties, for a short time at least, can be pushed to the back of your mind and will not compromise your safety.

What I suggest is a simple commentary system. As you move through your daily life, you give yourself a detailed, mental running commentary of everything that is happening around you. Obviously I am not advocating that you should do this every second of every day as you still need to interact with friends and concentrate on work.

To begin with, I suggest you practise it every time you go out into the public domain, which is, in most situations, when you are at your most vulnerable.

CHAPTER FIFTEEN

The commentary must be fluid, not dwelling too long on any one aspect, but it must also be as detailed as possible. Because you are doing it mentally, it is far quicker than talking about it. Come up with a set system for describing people and try always to do it in the same order. It does not really matter what order it goes in. but you need to get in their general physical appearance: height, build, skin colour, hair colour and style, distinguishing marks and then clothing. It helps if you start from the bottom or the top and work your way to the other end: that way you miss nothing. It does not matter which end you start from, but try and do it the same way every time as you move from person to person.

For instance, if you see a man waiting at the newsagents across the street from your office, you should not just register his presence, register his *appearance* too. Even though, a split second later, you have moved on and are in your office getting on with your day, the description you gave that man will remain in your subconscious.

Now, it could be that the man standing there was entirely innocent and had a legitimate reason for being there. This will be the case ninety nine times out of a hundred. But let's just say, on this one occasion, that this man is there for some sinister reason.

If you go into town at lunch time and, entering the public domain once more you "switch your commentary on" you will describe the people around you using the same system.

This morning you told yourself, *"There is a man stood outside the newsagents, he is tall and slim, he looks about 40 and has blond hair. He is wearing a black hoodie, blue jeans and white Nike trainers."*

So what would happen if a man was standing outside your favourite lunchtime haunt and, because you are switched on, he falls into your commentary with your usual system of description:

"There is a man stood outside the coffee shop, he is tall and

CHAPTER FIFTEEN

slim, he looks about 40 and has blond hair. He is wearing a black hoodie, blue jeans and white Nike trainers."

Even though, after seeing him this morning, you dismissed him, your personal system for describing people has just triggered the memory because what you told yourself was *exactly* the same as before. It could be mere coincidence, but you can now make a mental note to see if this person turns up again.

I have used a single person as an example here, but it could just as well be a group (where the description of them all taken together, as well as that of individual members can trigger a memory) or a vehicle parked somewhere. As long as you are paying attention and doing your mental commentary, anomalies should jump out at you.

It is extremely difficult to be truly nondescript. Everyone is distinctive. Even the ones with what is termed as average height and average build, with instantly forgettable conservative hairstyle and colour, will have something about them. The trick is attention to detail. Nothing, no matter how small, should be overlooked. In fact it is often the small, seemingly insignificant details that can be the most telling. Few people think to change the way they walk, for instance, and that can be as distinctive a character trait as a vivid hair colour.

The commentary system can also be used when you are driving your car. In fact, many advanced driving instructors adopt the method when teaching their students to observe the road and its environs. It will make you a better driver and less likely to be caught unawares.

On the subject of vehicles, it would be best if you do the same thing for them as you have done for the people that you see. Come up with a quick means of describing them so that you can log them and move on. Make, model and colour are all good and this can be backed up with the registration number. If you are not familiar with the makes of the various cars, simply log the colour and part of the

CHAPTER FIFTEEN

registration number. Anything that means you will recognise it if you see it again. It may have a distinctive rust patch, dent or window sticker. Anything that can be of use should be included.

Remember, whether you are driving or on foot, the observations must be constant and cover the full 360 degrees around you as the world is fluid and will be changing constantly. Do not linger on any aspect to the expense of others. Train yourself to take a mental snapshot and move on. The laws of survival in a city are the same as the ones in the wild. Concentrating too much on one person could blind you to their associates who are flanking you whilst you are distracted. Be aware of things going on around you, but do not get pulled into any one aspect of it unless it is absolutely necessary. Do not merely limit it to people and vehicles, try to see *everything*.

Eventually, you will find that you do not have to make a conscious effort to instigate the commentary. It will become something that your mind does on its own - you may not even register you are doing it any more. It will only become apparent when some anomaly occurs, such as seeing the same person twice as described above.

If you have a like-minded friend, use the commentary system to test each other on awareness of the things around you. It does not just have to be descriptions of cars and people, it could be the time on the church clock, or the breed of dog that just walked past. If you have to look to check, you lose a point and the one who loses the most points by the end of the week has to buy the coffees on Friday lunchtime. It is a fun and easy thing to do and will increase your awareness no end.

Remember however that when you are checking people out this could be misconstrued. In our culture staring at someone can be seen as merely rude, or it can mean an expression of interest, or even a challenge. Be mindful of this and make it a priority to speed up your assessments of people. Be aware of the buildings and parked vehicles around you - the reflections in their windows and

CHAPTER FIFTEEN

metallic surfaces can be an excellent surveillance tool. If you do think you are seeing the same person for the third time that day, get yourself across the street and use the reflection in the shop window to get a better look at your quarry.

(Bear in mind though, that you should be careful which shop you appear to be browsing in!)

Chapter 16

Routine

Some people are sticklers for routine and cannot function without it. Others find even the concept of routine too confining. The truth is, some form of routine is essential in order for us to function in modern society. Even VIPs under close protection still have a set schedule to meet and, although they may vary their routes to and from certain places, they always have to be there at certain places and times. These are times when awareness is heightened. If this is the only consistent part of their routine, it is the one a potential assassin would look at first.

Fortunately, the majority of people are not likely to be targeted by assassins anytime soon and, for the sake of efficiency, routines are an essential part of life. Whether it involves getting the children to school on time or taking part in a structured learning process, such as venturing out to attend a prearranged class, the fact that you have to be at a set place for a set time necessitates some form of structure to what you are doing.

As long as you are mindful and have trained your mind through your commentary, you will be aware of your surroundings and the people in it as you go about your routine. You will most likely see the same people every day, whether they are strangers waiting with you at a bus stop, fellow parents dropping children off at school or

CHAPTER SIXTEEN

the barista at the coffee shop you always call at, the same faces and situations will crop up.

Now, it might be that such a routine makes you complacent and lulls you into a false sense of security. You might find that the commentary training is getting boring and predictable, but as I said in the previous chapter, once you have trained your mind to consciously run through the commentary, it will not be long before your mind does it automatically. The beauty of having the same routine day in and day out is that as soon as your commentary notes something that is not a normal part of your routine, your brain will flag it up instantly. You will immediately realise that there is an anomaly and you can then assess the threat, if any, that this new development poses.

People do this all the time and do not realise it. Have you ever come home from work and seen a car parked on your street which you know does not belong to any of your neighbours? You may have been preoccupied thinking about your tea, or your plans for that evening, but this is intruded upon, without any conscious effort from you, by the appearance of the car. This is the kind of trigger that you can cultivate with mindful commentary and a set routine.

The beauty of routine is that you can streamline your commentary. This does not mean that you are being any less thorough, or that you can become complacent. It merely means that there will be aspects of your environment which are constant. If you have already memorised a description of a car or a person, all you need to do is augment this by confirming your initial assessment with a quick glance when you encounter them on future occasions. This sounds complicated and seems as if it will require a conscious effort *not* to engage in a full commentary, but the truth is that your brain will do it for you, probably without you realising it.

So your routine every morning is the same. You are up, you are ready and you are out for the usual time, travelling to work or school by whatever means you prefer.

CHAPTER SIXTEEN

Now, hopefully this can go on, day in and day out, indefinitely. There is also the unfortunate chance that it may not. You may notice that a stranger is taking an unhealthy interest in you, an intimidating gang has taken up residence on the street corner which forms part of your route to work or that the same occupied vehicle is parked on your street a few days running.

Now, it may be that the stranger is merely wanting to pluck up the courage to engage you in innocent conversation, that the gang of children are just a bunch of essentially nice kids suffering from terminal boredom and the car belongs to a new friend of your neighbour picking them up for work. But the truth is that whether the anomaly is cause for concern or not cannot be ascertained without pushing your luck and playing into their hands.

Remember, ego has no part of self protection. If you spot an anomaly and it makes you uncomfortable, that feeling was created by your mind for a reason. The age-old instinct for self preservation is kicking in and now is the time to vary your routine.

I would suggest that you do not go for a full revamp of absolutely everything that you do to get from A to B, and it may not be possible for you to do that anyway. Whichever part of your routine that anomaly was noted in is this one you need to address first.

For instance, if the anomaly was a creepy bloke watching you getting on or off your bus, you could catch a bus at a different time, or get off at a different stop. If it was someone who always seemed to be in a certain place at a certain time, vary the place or vary the time, or both.

By only altering the one aspect of your routine, it means your hard-earned commentary from the rest of your route can stay and the new part would get the full conscious treatment. If the anomaly follows your new routine then I would suggest that you may have a problem and may wish to take it further. (By this I mean engaging the authorities, not fronting the person up.)

Now, as I mentioned for VIPs, there will be some aspects of your

CHAPTER SIXTEEN

routine which you cannot vary. Your children will attend the same school regardless of the time you get them there and you will always have the same workplace and the same home. If someone is really interested in you, this is the fixed point they need to observe you. These are locations of *heightened* awareness. You should already be extremely aware due to your commentary and being rooted in the moment, but these are the areas where it would be best, even after you have trained your commentary and it is second nature, to bring it to the forefront of your consciousness again and engage it the same way you did as a beginner. Besides the fact that it is always good to get back to basics and sharpen your skills, these are the times during your routine when you will be at your most vulnerable. You are approaching work, with the Monday morning blues and, although you haven't thought about it all weekend, you suddenly think of the list of things to do stuck on your monitor, or you are rushing towards home through the rain and the thought of getting in and having a warm drink and something to eat will pop into your head. With the best will in the world, there will be times when things like this will happen. Knowing your weak spots is an essential tool in staying on point. It will give you an indication of when you need to elevate your awareness even more.

Chapter 17

Making yourself a harder target

For those who are unfamiliar with the expression, "target hardening" means exactly that - making yourself so hard a target that any potential attackers see you as too much hassle to take on.

This does not necessarily mean that they think you can take them in a fight. Predators such as these are cowards deep down and believe in safety in numbers. Get most of them one on one and their true colours would be revealed. Get them in a gang and, dependent upon its size, watch their "courage" grow exponentially.

Whilst a would-be attacker is scanning the people around him looking for a potential victim he is in a relatively low-risk stage, provided he does not arouse suspicion. His problem arises when he is actually committing the offence. He wants it to be over and done with as soon as possible to minimise the risk of injury, witnesses and capture. For these reasons he will instinctively single out the easiest "mark" he can find. He may not even register his thought processes, but will look first for people who are alone. He will look for those he perceives to be weaker than he is (this becomes moot where greater numbers are involved, see the above re group "bravery") and those who appear distracted. He will look for overt signs of prosperity. The location will also play a factor. This list is not exhaustive, but illustrates the many factors that can come into play.

CHAPTER SEVENTEEN

Looking for people who are alone

There are occasions when multiple victims have been selected and singled out, usually when offenders are in greater numbers or have some physical advantage over their prey, such as two older boys picking on two younger ones because they want their bikes, but the majority of victims will be people travelling on their own.

If you need to travel alone, there is nothing that can be done about that, but it needs to be borne in mind that this may make you more of a potential target. Hopefully, after we have run through some of the other factors, this will not be so much of an issue.

People who are perceived to be weaker

This does not just apply to the people the attacker thinks are weaker than they are, it also means that they will look for the weakest person amongst all the potential victims they consider.

I appreciate that some people are more physically intimidating than others through their height and build and general overall presence and would be quickly deleted from the list of potentials, but it will then fall to the remainder, the group of people with average height and build. This means most people, so the pickings can be very rich indeed.

The way you walk and generally carry yourself can be a great leveller. If you are practising your commentary and are in the moment you will be alert to everything around you. Hopefully you would register the presence of your would-be attacker long before a potential approach and, if he is observed, that is one plus on your column. He may think you are too hard a target.

Similarly, it may be that there is a group which has separated in the general area. If you spot them all, and they *know* they have been spotted (again, without issuing subliminal challenges, just showing that you are aware), they will move on.

CHAPTER SEVENTEEN

You may not feel confident – indeed as you walk along you may be absolutely terrified - but this fear has to be displayed for the attacker to register it. Project confidence through your gait and demeanour, walk confidently and stand tall. Most people tend to slouch slightly when they walk. Someone standing tall and oozing confidence would make you stand out in the crowd, but not for the reasons the attacker wants.

If you are carrying a bag of any description, keep it close to your body. If it has a zip opener, make sure the tab of your zip is towards the front of your body, so that no-one can open with without you seeing or being aware. If it has a flap, or side pockets, carry it with the flap or pockets resting against your body. If you need to carry a laptop and are fearful of losing it, do not carry it in a laptop case but use a nondescript bag which will not give any indication as to the contents.

Sometimes, an offender may bring along a weapon with which to intimidate the attacker. This does not necessarily mean they intend to use it. Nine times out of ten it is the *threat* of the weapon that is sufficient for them to commit the offence. The presence of the weapon can change the target selection slightly, but it is the same formula being followed. Make yourself a harder target by bringing all these factors into play and they will instinctively move on to another potential victim. We are hoping to avoid the confrontation a long while before it gets to the weapon drawing phase.

People who appear distracted

People who are distracted and preoccupied will be perceived by the offender as good potential victims, particularly for a "blitz" attack whereby they intend to snatch a bag and run, or blindside them.

Sadly, in this day and age, many people walk the streets distracted by modern technology. Mobile phones and iPods are in almost constant use. I am afraid that if you are in public and are

CHAPTER SEVENTEEN

not in a place of relative safety, the use of electronic devices is unnecessarily risky.

If your phone rings whilst you are walking, do not take it out and answer it in the street. Step into a shop and answer it, then watch the street through the shop window or, better still, let it register as a missed call and then deal with it when you reach your destination. Even the use of Bluetooth or an iPod is fraught with danger. Whilst you have your conscious thoughts divided between your environment and the sounds going into your ear you are not fully aware of your surroundings and are increasing your potential as a victim.

Speak to your colleagues and associates and tell them that should they ever ring whilst you are out and about, there is a chance you will not answer the phone. It is an extreme rarity that answering a call needs to take precedence over your personal safety. I'm sorry but many calls perceived to be emergencies or "a matter of life and death" are nothing of the kind. Relative safety to either answer or return the call is likely to be a couple of minutes away. It is up to you, but, if you take self-protection seriously, you will not make yourself a potential target by being distracted by a phone call or digitised music.

I own an iPod, but I rarely listen to it away from its base station because I am rarely in a position where I can safely do so. If you absolutely need your music, wait until you are sitting on the bus/train or in the coffee shop and, whilst you are listening to it, keep your eyes peeled. Watch the other passengers getting on, watch the entrance to the shop and the customers. It is imperative that you do not appear distracted (even though, technically, you are).

Whilst on the subject of iPods, one thing I find really risky is wearing them whilst running. There is absolutely nothing wrong with wearing your iPod whilst working out in the gym or on the treadmill, but as soon as you venture into the public domain it puts you at unnecessary risk.

If you find that you cannot get through a run without some

music, then I would suggest that you find some other form of exercise, because you are not enjoying the run itself and the music is a means to get through it. The majority of runners do it for the sheer thrill of running and take in their surroundings as part of the pleasure of the run. There are even adventure holidays for runners which give them the opportunity to run through areas of natural beauty. There is always something going on for you to see. Your internal dialogue needs to be taken up with commentary, not music.

When you are running with iPod buds in your ears, you are distracted. There is the risk of traffic if you run in built-up areas and there is the risk of being distracted and alone if you are trail running. Yes, you might be able to outrun the obese pervert who comes at you out of the bushes wearing nothing but a smile, but if you run the same route every time, all he has to do is wait.

Please do not think I am trying to make you paranoid or I'm trying to spoil your fun, but I want people to move away from the concept that bad things only happen to other people.

Some time ago, there was a spate of thefts at a supermarket near where I live. Women pushing trolleys loaded with shopping had put their handbags on top of the shopping for the short walk to the car. The offender (who was eventually caught) ran up, snatched the handbag, and ran. How simple is that? And, equally, how simple would it be to avoid that happening?

The truth is that the victims never expected such an audacious crime. It never entered their heads that something like this could happen because it was so unusual, but happen it did.

Whilst I am in no way intending to be derogatory towards the victims, or to trivialise their ordeal, not being distracted and being aware of the surroundings and the potential risks could have taken them out of the running as a potential victim.

Take a look at the factors that had to come into play for the offence to happen. When you consider how many people exit and enter a supermarket every day, and the fact that the offence was

CHAPTER SEVENTEEN

only committed against a handful, some other factors must have come into play regarding victim selection.

Because they are targeting handbags, the potential victim must have been a woman. This does not necessarily mean a woman alone, but a woman had to be present for the intended goods to be available. The size and intimidation factors or the presence of spouses and friends do not come into play here because no physical confrontation is sought. But the presence of others with their chosen victim would still have been a factor guiding their selection.

Secondly, the handbag had to be in the trolley, on top of the shopping and within easy reach. If the woman had the bag over her shoulder, or had the strap looped around her hand, they would not have got it.

Thirdly, for this kind of sneak attack, the offender would want to remain unnoticed until the last possible moment and then flee the scene as fast as possible.

Now, if a lone female exits the store and our offender see that she has her bag over her shoulder, fastened, with the end that opens towards the front of her body so that no one can open the bag without her knowledge, and she checks her environment and is totally aware, then she would be too hard a target for our offender and she would be struck off the victim list without ever knowing she had been on it.

Similarly, before you leave the sanctity of the store, have your car keys in your hand. This will negate the need to distract yourself from your environment by having to rummage through your pockets or handbag when you reach your car.

Nowadays, crime prevention campaigns are catching up about protecting PIN numbers when visiting an ATM, but there is also a need for general awareness regarding the card and the cash when the transaction is complete. I have seen people turn away from the ATM with a wad of notes in their hand openly counting it as they walk away. Do I need to elaborate on the risks inherent in this kind of distraction? I could go on with these kind of examples but the truth is, they would all be variations on a theme.

Overt signs of prosperity

I am still amazed when I read reports that people have left their sat nav or phone on general display in their car and then had it broken into. There have been hundreds of anti crime campaigns over the years decrying this sort of oversight, but there are not too many about pedestrians having their wealth on display.

I wish people could wear what they want without fear of harassment, reprisal or opportunistic crime, but the sad truth is, they cannot.

It is purely a matter of choice whether you openly display your new iPhone, Rolex or jewellery. But please bear in mind that drawing the attention of the world in general to your prized acquisitions, will also draw the attention of the criminals.

Locations

Most of the time, we have a choice in what route we can take to get from A to B. You know the areas around where you live, you know the parts which are "unsavoury" and the parts which are "exclusive" (there are more of the former, and less of the latter where I live!)

Although it is not uncommon for crimes to be committed in a relatively crowded place, they are not the ideal location for crime due to the high volume of witnesses and the general profusion of CCTV coverage. You will be aware of quieter areas where you live. These are areas of heightened risk. If, despite your best efforts, you do not identify your would-be attackers and then enter a quiet area with no one around, chances are that is where it will happen.

It is best to identify and avoid these areas wherever possible.

CHAPTER SEVENTEEN

Similarly, if you need to travel to a place you have never visited before, do some groundwork before your trip. Look the place up on the internet, look through news articles on crime in that area, check out the website of the local police, even ring them for advice on no-go areas, and generally learn as much as you can before you go.

Do not rely too much on your satellite navigation system. It may guide you unerringly to your destination, but will not take into account the kinds of areas it will take you through and, when you reach your destination, be careful where you park your car. The nice leafy street you parked it on amidst the afternoon sunshine may be a totally different place when the sun goes down.

When you approach your car, have your keys in your hand well in advance. Do not be distracted rummaging for them while standing beside your vehicle. If someone steals your keys a street away, they would have a hard time finding the car to go with them. If you're standing there rummaging through your pockets you are going to lose your keys and your car.

One other thing before we leave this section. Offenders have no morals. Their standards are not your standards and you would be amazed at the lengths they would go to when pursuing their craft. Never think, for instance, "I'll be ok walking with my daughter in the pushchair, no-one would attack a man/woman with a baby", because you would be dead wrong. There have been cases where offenders held a knife to a baby's throat in order to force the mother to capitulate to their demands (and this was in the UK).

Desperation can play a part where opportunistic offenders are concerned. Many only take this risk because they are stealing to feed a habit. It is a habit that ultimately consumes their every waking moment, where abstinence from their chosen vice causes intense pain and depression. All they can think about is their next fix, so their moral compass becomes redundant in their pursuit of their goal.

I had this discussion with someone once and he shifted the argument, stating that the addict shouldn't have started on the drugs in the first place and that it was their own doing. In the sphere of self-protection, their past history is irrelevant. What matters is the here and now and the fact that they pose a threat. Espousing moral dictates is moot. They are what they are and that is what you have to deal with.

Please do not fall into the trap of thinking that everyone shares your standards and ethos. They do not and I would not want the realisation of this fact to be revealed through someone becoming a victim of violent crime.

Remember, all we are trying to do is make ourselves too difficult a target for a would-be attacker to deal with. While the above list is not exhaustive, it covers some of the factors and sets out general principles which can be adhered to and adapted to other situations.

Chapter 18

Identifying areas of heightened risk

We have already touched on these areas earlier, but I wanted to spend a little time talking about these and how to prepare for them. In the last chapter we talked about target hardening in relation to opportunistic street crime. But what if you had been singled out for reasons other than the victim indicators we have mentioned?

What if your ex decides that they do not want the relationship to end and, in their mind, it is still going on? What if the co-worker who avoids you because he is shy is actually bottling up lustful emotions for you and lacks the social skills to approach attraction the way others do? People have been murdered merely because their physical appearance is reminiscent of the killer's abusive parent. The motives for crime can sometimes seem irrational and obscure to all but those who commit the offence.

Remember, we are working on the premise that bad things can and do happen and there's no reason they cannot happen to you.

Sit down with a notepad and pen and make a list of everywhere you are required to be at a set place and time. This includes work, school, church, scheduled evening classes (both for you and for anyone you take to these classes) and social groups (Weightwatchers, religious groups, running clubs, your dojo etc.). You also need to include the times you leave and return to your home.

CHAPTER EIGHTEEN

Next, add on the places you go as a matter of routine, where arrival at that day and time is not required *per se*, it is just the way you like to do things. For instance, you may like to do your shopping at the same store every Saturday afternoon. My wife meets her friend for a coffee at the same venue every Friday after they have picked the girls up from school. You may favour an early morning run, or go swimming before work. Anything that has fallen into the realms of routine needs to be on the list.

In addition, if you are a parent, you need to list the routines and requirements of your children too. Unsavoury as it may sound, children can be targeted, and their safety is your responsibility.

Unless you are incarcerated, or in hibernation, you should have quite a long and comprehensive list. Every single item on that list is an area of *heightened risk*. They are all points where a potential offender can guarantee that they will see you or meet you.

If he or she first saw you at two o'clock on Saturday afternoon in Morrison's, they will return to Morrison's at that time and day in order to try and see you again. If you always take your children swimming at six o'clock on a Wednesday to the local leisure centre, then this is another point of contact, and so on.

The thing is, seeing these people every time you attend these locations can very easily become part of the routine and, as long as they keep their distance you may not register a threat. This is where the use of mindfulness and the commentary come into play. If you are totally aware, any nefarious approach on their part will be scuppered before it can begin. They may try to use conversation in order to slide under your radar but, as long as you are polite, there are no rules that state you have to engage in something that makes you uncomfortable just because you think it is "socially acceptable" to do so.

If you suddenly find the same person cropping up at more than one of your routine destinations, then this crossover could constitute a higher level of threat. It could be pure coincidence, but

CHAPTER EIGHTEEN

that person could know more about your routines than they should.

I am not suggesting that you become totally paranoid and sociopathic. There are a lot of really nice people out there who may just be looking for friendship or a new relationship. It is a matter for you and your instincts what approach you take. Trust your instincts though, some risks just are not worth taking.

If you do decide to take the person up on that offer of a drink or date, *you* set the time and venue. If they offer to come and pick you up, politely decline and arrange to meet them there.

This effectively negates the creation of a new area of heightened risk. It stops them finding out where you live, it cuts down the risk of getting in their car (effectively putting you entirely at their mercy) and it means you can choose a venue that is safe, not one selected by them that they may have already formulated a plan around beforehand. If, by the end of the night, you decide that it is not what you want, they will know nothing more about you than they already do (unless you tell them your life story during your conversations, but that is a matter for you) and when you go your separate ways things will return to being as they were, although you may consider a variance in your routine concerning the venue where you actually met them for the first time.

If your date involves the consumption of alcoholic beverages, never leave your drink unattended and, if you are holding a bottle, keep your thumb over the opening in between drinks.

The main problem with these situations arises from the fact that some predators are extremely clever at hiding their true persona and by the time potential victims realise they are in over their heads, it is too late.

Try not to let healthy self-protection become unhealthy paranoia, and try to find the balance in between. If your date is one of the legitimate "nice people", of which there are many, they will not mind taking things steady and will not mind your caution. If they do, that is a warning signal right there.

CHAPTER EIGHTEEN

Do not let personal aspects of your date lower your guard. A person's chosen occupation is not always an indicator of what kind of person they are. There are abusive and corrupt people in all walks of life. Similarly, there are people who are not what they look like. Some people may be huge and covered in tattoos but are surprisingly erudite. It is a common misconception that all fighters are unintelligent. Many are extremely well read and possess a level of discipline that few others could aspire to. The paradox of martial arts and fighting is that, in most cases, the artists leave their aggression in the gym or dojo and as a result are much calmer and more tolerant than those who get no exercise and have no outlet for their stress.

Obviously, there are exceptions to every rule, but I just wanted to illustrate that books cannot be judged by their covers.

If you regularly visit certain places, but do not have to go on a set date or at a set time, vary your visits as discussed earlier, but merely being aware that they are areas of heightened risk should have a positive effect on your mindful commentary.

If you have to be somewhere regularly at a certain day and time there may be nothing you can do about it. Again, you can vary your routes or your modes of travel. You could ask your spouse to take the children for a change, or you could *both* take them. I once dealt with a case of harassment where the man would not let the victim bring an end to their relationship. Whilst she was single she had non-stop problems from this aloof, annoying, narcissist. He was arrested a couple of times under the Harassment Act but kept on going regardless. Then, one day, the victim found herself a new boyfriend and our offender never bothered her again. The fact is, showing any as yet unknown predators that you are in a relationship can be a form of target hardening in itself.

So, having identified your areas of heightened risk, think about how to target-harden your attendance there if you need to. Once

CHAPTER EIGHTEEN

again, you should not fall into the paranoid camp and vary your routines constantly, this would just cause you undue stress.

All you need to do is look at your list, at each area of heightened risk, and come up with a few plans to vary your routine if required. I know I have said it before, but just registering that they are areas of heightened risk is a start. Coming up with plans proactively is far better than trying to plan on the fly. Remember, one of the things we are doing is to try and protect ourselves by removing unnecessary worries from our mind. Plan ahead, write the plans down and take the anxiety out of your head, where it can clutter your thinking.

Chapter 19

At home

Everyone needs a place where they can relax and unwind. For the majority of people, this means home. People who avoid going home and find their relaxation and distraction elsewhere have deeper problems which fall outside the scope of this text and should speak to someone (I am not joking this time, if you have a problem with going home, which should be your place of safety, please ask yourself why).

Now, as you read this text, it would be very easy to feel I am implying that you should be constantly on your guard and jumping at every shadow, but the truth is that the more you practise mindfulness and, therefore, *zanshin* and *mushin*, and follow the suggestions we have already discussed, the more they will become second nature. Because you are teaching yourself to stay rooted in the moment, your concentration will be the same throughout your day, giving you a natural state of constant vigilance which does not feel forced or paranoid.

When you go home to your "place of safety", this mindfulness should continue, as it should be more than just a tool for self-protection. Utilising mindful routines within the home can afford you the same level of protection that mindfulness gives you in the public domain.

For instance, every night, before I retire to bed, I check that the

CHAPTER NINETEEN

front door is locked. I then walk through to the kitchen, turning the lights off as I go, put some food out for the constantly ravenous pair of cats who live with us (I cannot call them pets as they are actually higher in the pecking order than I am, as is our rabbit) and then check that the back door is locked before going upstairs.

I do this as a routine. Sometimes I am extremely tired when I do it, but not so tired that if I checked a door and found it unlocked, I would not think to lock it. Routines like this are simple and easy to follow and, once you have done them a few times, they become second nature. It is also good if your partner goes through the same ritual, so you make doubly sure that the house is secure.

During the summer months, I always keep an eye on which windows, if any, we open during the course of the day, and these are also checked, even though I know they will be locked as soon as they are closed. Also, there is always a peak in the trend of "sneak in" burglaries during the summer months where people leave open doors unattended and the offenders simply walk in, grab what they can, and make good their escape before the occupant knows they were there. If you have a door open because the weather is warm, make sure you close it when you leave the room. It takes mere seconds to open and close a door, so if you are saying to yourself that you cannot be bothered, on your head be it.

It is best, if you are to have these routines, to put them to some kind of system. For instance, if you are leaving the house and want to make sure everything is switched off and the house is being left secure, conduct your search systematically, room by room, starting from the furthest point and working your way towards the exit - that way you make sure you do not miss a room.

When it starts to get dark and you need to put your lights on, close the blinds or curtains. It amazes me how many people leave their lives, and the contents of their houses, on display during the winter evenings by having all their lights blazing and all their curtains open. This is also worth bearing in mind in the morning as people

CHAPTER NINETEEN

tend to think that crimes will be committed in the evenings. Do not take anything for granted.

We are fortunate enough to have two cars. My wife parks hers on our driveway and I park mine at the front of the house. I actually park it so that my windows are parallel with the front of the house, slightly off centre, opposite where the door is situated. This means that, if I am upstairs and someone knocks on the door, I can glance out of the bedroom window and see my visitor reflected in the car windows. The use of reflections is an excellent tool and should be drawn upon wherever possible.

Mobile phones are mobile for a reason, so that we can take them wherever we go. Yes, I know that sounds inane and obvious, but how many people mislay their mobile phones at home? My wife does it to such an extent that her friend bought her a mobile phone holder, so she would always know where the phone was.

Put your mobile in the same place when you are downstairs, and have a place for it upstairs. Get into the habit of keeping them close at hand, not necessarily in the same room or on your person, just easily accessible, and always in the same place wherever possible. This means you can find them in the dark, or if your vision is limited, for example by smoke. The same can be said for your keys. Burglaries happen today where homes are targeted because the occupants own a nice car. The actual invasion of the home is merely in order to steal the car keys. Always know where your keys are, do not leave them in an obvious place, and *never* leave them in the door lock.

On the subject of darkness and limited visual capability, get to know your way around your house without having to look. You can keep your hands out to feel for walls etc, but getting to know the layout so you can navigate through your house in complete darkness gives you an enormous advantage in the unfortunate event that you encounter an intruder. It will give you more confidence moving around the house at night or during a power cut, and will mean that

CHAPTER NINETEEN

you no longer hammer your shin or your toes on things you should know are there and waking up the rest of the household.

A lot of people have a plan for looking after their families in the event of a fire, and this is an excellent thing to do, but you and your family should also have a plan for what to do if someone gets into your home. Do not give yourself or the rest of your family nightmares. Chances are you will hear any intruders before the children do, and it is merely a case of making sure everyone is safe and accounted for. Get the children into your room or you go into theirs, but make sure the mobile phone goes with you.

You may have encountered this phenomenon or you may not, but usually, in a household with children, the mother will stir at the first signs of a sound from the child's bedroom. Whilst the father may sleep through the child waking up, he will stir at the first sign of a sound that shouldn't be there, like the creak of a floorboard or a cupboard closing downstairs.

Remember that self protection is about target hardening and making yourself a less vulnerable member of the herd so the predator puts you firmly in the "too hard to do" column. With this in mind, and extended to the target hardening of your home, there are a myriad of different crime prevention devices on the market. At the very least, you should make sure that all your doors and windows have stout locks (and use them) and, if possible invest in an alarm. Unless you have been specifically targeted, making your house look just too difficult will force them to look for something easier. If you contact your local police station, they should have a crime prevention officer who can advise you about home security.

I know some people keep weapons to hand in their houses, and I am not going to enter into an ethical debate about the pros and cons of facing off with intruders and the physical side of the actual point of conflict was handled in part one of this text, but what I will say is that leaving a baseball bat beside your door at the very least arms an intruder as they come in and, at best, you could find your intruder in between you and your "weapon".

CHAPTER NINETEEN

If you do find yourself in the unfortunate situation where someone is in your house, the best weapon you can use is to raise the alarm, so keep your phone handy, make sure everyone you care about is accounted for, and call the authorities. As I said, whether you choose to search your house and potentially engage the intruder is a matter for you but personally, I would want to *at least* place myself in between them and my family.

I could go on and on about what to do and what not to do if someone gets into your house, but the truth is that we all react in different ways and it is very much up to the individual. Remember though, that what you *say* you would do now in the cold light of day may be completely at odds with what you would actually do at four in the morning when you are half asleep. This portion of the text is more about mindful target hardening, developing *zanshin* and *mushin* and establishing routines and systems within the home so that you are doing everything you can to deter those that would harm you or steal your property.

Conclusion: Part 1

A brief, pragmatic look at the twenty guiding principles

This text is about making your practice of traditional karate more practical, but as illustrated through the latter portions of the book, this goes beyond merely making the physical techniques more practical.

I mentioned the "Twenty Guiding Principles of Karate" when we discussed stances (principle seventeen), and *karate ni sente nashi* is actually principle number two. So we will now go through the remaining eighteen principles and apply them to a modern setting. The principles are taken directly from *The Twenty Guiding Principles of Karate* by Gichin Funakoshi, published by Kodansha International (2003).

This will, I hope, serve to convey that what Master Funakoshi felt constituted a *karateka* is as relevant today as it was then. Some of it reiterates text which I have already covered and I make no apologies for this reiteration - it needs hammering home.

Do not forget that Karate-do begins and ends with Rei (principle one).

It is significant that this first principle speaks of the *Do,* the way of karate. This is obviously written from the viewpoint that both the physical and emotional development of the *karateka* was seen as a high priority. I see this as extending much further than a token bow as you enter and leave the dojo and a bow to your opponent.

This is, fundamentally, about respect. I am not talking about a respect borne out of awe or fear that may be shown to a fighter (respect borne of fear is not respect anyway, it is fear manifested as subjugation). Everything around you demands a certain level of respect by the mere fact that it *exists*. The planet itself, the flora, fauna and the humans, should all receive that fundamental level of respect.

One of the best bits of advice a police officer ever gave me about entering a potentially volatile situation was to appear calm and respectful. If the need arises, you can then escalate. It is far better to come into a situation at ground level and ascend to twenty thousand feet if you have to, than to enter it at that height and have to descend to ground level after damage is done. This doesn't just apply to volatile situations - it can apply to every encounter in your life, no matter how mundane.

Principle two, as stated, is *karate ni sente nashi*, which was given a chapter of its own.

Karate stands on the side of justice (principle three).

Ah! If only this was true. We can all think of examples of *karateka* who have, shall we say, questionable moral rectitude. This is very much an individual thing, and, ironically, karate was seen as a main pursuit of the Yakuza at one time. A number of these principles interweave and, if you respect other people and their property as defined in principle one, following this one should be easy.

I cannot tell you how to behave, you would need to be guided by your own moral compass on that one. What I will say is this, you are reading this text as you want to make your traditional karate more pragmatic whilst not deviating from the way. This is one of the Way's guiding principles.

First know yourself, then know others (principle four).

The only person who really knows you is you. As stated in the section on ego, we all have a persona which we like to project out into the world and a way that we would like to be seen. It comes as a surprise to some that this is based on *your* perceptions of who you are, not those of other people, and what they think of you may not be what you wanted.

Once again, one of the hardest things in the world to do is take an *honest* look at yourself and the way you behave. Merely recognising your own flaws (to yourself, no-one else needs to know) and making a conscious effort to improve them will have a cathartic effect in itself.

Once you have dissected yourself, and discovered what makes you tick, it is far easier to gain tolerance and understanding for those around you. Everyone else has insecurities, worries and preoccupations which will dictate their moods and behaviour at any given time, no matter what persona they project to the world. By knowing yourself, you get to know others, and become more tolerant as a result.

Mentality over technique (principle five).

Your mind is the best weapon you have, though the mental side of martial arts has taken something of a back step these days in favour of the search for physical technique. Cultivate concentration, meditate, employ the tactics discussed in the section on *zanshin* and *mushin*. It is no accident that books like the *Art of War* and the *Book Of Five Rings* are used in the world of business as well as martial arts, or that many martial artists tend to enjoy and sometimes excel at chess and Go. They cultivate an analytical mind and they teach strategy that is not just for the "battlefield", but can also be applied to life. If you use your mind correctly, you will safely navigate past more violent situations than you get involved in. Impetuosity has no place in karate-do (as the *dojo-kun* clearly states.)

The mind must be set free (principle six).

Contrary to how it may first appear, this does not contradict principle five. I believe that what it being cited here is that the mind is something that you *use*. If you are not careful, you can *become* your mind and it can control you. As I stated in the section on *mushin*, having "no mind" is desirable in conflict, but *mushin* comes from the fact that a decision has been made, and it is time to get on with it and not to allow anything to distract you. Funakoshi makes reference to Zen in his text and there is a great deal of Buddhism in the short title to this principle. It basically says that there is only the present moment, so worrying about the past and future is futile. Employ the mind to resolve dilemmas in the here and now, once it is solved, the mind has to behave itself once again. Do not let your mind rule you, show it who's boss.

Calamity springs from carelessness (principle seven).

This pretty much speaks for itself. The majority of these principles focus on the correct cultivation of the mind, and this is no exception. Being mindful in everything you do (we are back to *zanshin* again) can ensure that you avoid pitfalls and problems throughout your day. Being preoccupied about work when you swing through a junction could lead to you cutting up a fellow motorist, followed by road rage and a violent scene, but if, once again, we talk about keeping rooted in the here and now and giving full focus to what we are currently doing, such calamities can be avoided.

Karate goes beyond the dojo (principle eight).

This is not a free licence to start brawling in the street. It implies that what you learn in the dojo about character and respect should not be left at the dojo door but carried with you into the rest of your life. Your training, if imparted correctly, can have an impact on your whole personality and this should be cultivated and adhered to even when you are away from the dojo.

Karate is a lifelong pursuit (principle nine).

I do not train, or execute my techniques, the same way I did twenty years ago. I am not physically capable of doing some of the things I did then. I recognise and accept that. I am, however, still training in karate.

There may be times during your life when you have to halt the physical training through injury or illness. This does not mean you have to abandon the philosophy. It is inevitable that your training and approach will change as time goes on, but once you are in, if you take what you are doing seriously, you are in it for life.

Apply the way of karate to all things, therein lies its beauty (principle ten).

The shrewdness of Funakoshi in his sales pitch to the Japanese people shines through in this principle. Obviously, he was not espousing the physical side of karate in this comment, he was very much rooted in the pursuit of the *do*.

Applying the same principles in real life as one does in the dojo, refraining from impetuosity, cultivating the same spirit of perseverance in all things as with your karate and upholding the precepts regarding honour and the treatment of others, are as relevant now as they were when first introduced (some would argue that these ideals are sadly lacking these days and a return to these concepts is more important than ever).

Karate is like boiling water, without heat it returns to its tepid state (principle eleven).

This concept applies to both the physical and spiritual side of training. Without constant physical training the techniques used become rusty, physical fitness reduces over time and the body becomes weak. Fitness is something that takes effort to gain, but can be lost quickly and easily.

It is exactly the same with the mental and spiritual side of the training. Without being constantly mindful of the way you conduct yourself, old, bad habits will return. If training the mind was easy, we would all be calm and controlled all the time. Sadly, this is not the case and the training of your mind is every bit as important as training your body, possibly more so.

Do not think of winning. Think, rather, of not losing (principle twelve).

At first glance, this has the look of a zen *koan*, as surely "winning" and "not losing" are one and the same, aren't they?

No, they are not. In order to "win", you have to throw yourself into the race. In order to "not lose", you do not even have to enter. Earlier, I mentioned that ego has no place in combat. If you could take ego out of the equation, the majority of fights would not take place. Ego destroys self control and leads people into situations that are extremely difficult to escape from. It is ego that gives rise to the desire to "win".

CONCLUSION: PART 1

If you are not ruled by your ego, you will not be drawn into conflict as easily and can therefore extricate yourself. You are not thinking of "winning". Get the mind set that if you let your ego get the better of you, then you "lose". Hence, think of "not losing" to your ego, rather than getting yourself into a situation where you need to think about winning.

In a physical sense, as Dalton so memorably quipped in *Roadhouse*, no-one ever wins a fight. If you are drawn into conflict, we are really into damage limitation. Serious physical injury arises from fights all over the world every day.

Concentrate on keeping yourself in one piece as much as possible. That means, in a real situation, if it reaches the point of resorting to the physical, think simply about the removal of threat. Be first, but be justified. Damage is not just physical, and neither is "loss".

Make adjustments according to your opponent (principle thirteen).

As I stated earlier, it is best if you hone weapons that will work regardless of your opponent's size and shape. (It is impossible to account for skill. Do not assume that someone cannot fight if they look out of shape - you may be in for a surprise). There are, however, other considerations. If your opponent is overweight, then his knees will be weaker as they are bearing so much weight. If he is long and lanky, go inside, if he's short and stocky, just the opposite. All this is easier said than done, of course, and my advice would be to hone the "catch all" weapons, but bear your opponent's physical attributes in mind.

CONCLUSION: PART 1

The outcome of a battle depends on how one handles emptiness and fullness (principle fourteen).

For this principle, Funakoshi borrows heavily from Sun Tzu and relates this to battlefield tactics. Our concerns, for the purposes of this text, are on a much smaller scale. They basically revolve around making the decision to yield or advance. I think this links in with the principles of Aikido and Judo, allowing your opponent to use their own strength against them. I was once training with a Tai Chi *sifu* who believed in the same concept.

It is very easy when training in traditional karate to become a little too tense, rigid and over-dependent on a misinterpretation of *kime* (mistaking it for tension when it is actually the *focus* applied to your technique). Experiment with going "soft" and yielding, and pay attention to your breath too. Holding your breath, or fast shallow breathing, are common problems in stressful situations and learning to control your breathing will greatly assist you.

Tai Chi is not just practised in a slow and relaxed manner for its health benefits. The *sifu* I trained with told me that performing the techniques slowly with relaxation was still used in the combative side of the art as it trained the muscles to remain relaxed through a full range of movement. The speed and subsequent power he could generate through relaxation and the correct application of breathing and body mechanics was phenomenal.

Think of the opponent's hands and feet as swords (principle fifteen).

In the world of the samurai, where wielding the sword was elevated to an art form, the concept of "one strike, one kill" was the ultimate aspiration. When you faced your opponent, the ultimate skill would be to draw your sword and strike him down before he could draw his. As soon as your opponent's sword left its scabbard, your chances of injury would go through the roof.

From an "empty hand" point of view, this concept translates nicely when the opponent's weapons are likened to a dangerous blade. If your opponent has a chance to "draw" or "deploy" them anywhere near you, you could be in trouble.

This returns us to the pre-emptive strike. As soon as you have the reasonable and honest belief that you are in danger, you strike. You don't wait for your opponent to "show" his weapons. Also, just like the samurai, your attack should be simple and decisive. Overly complicated techniques are not to be trusted when you are under undue stress.

When you step beyond your own gate, you face a million enemies (principle sixteen).

The obvious interpretation of this is that of *zanshin* and the necessity to cultivate awareness of your surroundings and the people in it. This takes little explanation. There are also, however, the enemies *within*, which must be faced. All day, every day, pitfalls will arise and you will be given ample time to practise the mental aspects of the *do*. Reigning in your anger, coping with stress and killing the ego *no matter how others treat you* takes constant discipline. Seeing the inner problems as *enemies* is a sound way to put them into context.

Principle seventeen was covered earlier when we discussed mobility.

Perform kata exactly; actual combat is another matter (principle eighteen).

It is interesting that Funakoshi thought to add this concept, as his master, Yasutsune Itosu, tinkered with older "established" *kata* to create the *Heian* series, and several techniques were altered to make the art more palatable for schoolchildren to practise. Actually, I don't think hypocrisy was at work here, despite what the principle might imply, and I do not think it was the stances and techniques he was talking about either. I think he was talking about the ritualistic trappings which can surround the practice of kata.

The strange *kamae* (the *Bassai* kata spring to mind) are more likely misinterpreted engagement techniques, and the rituals of *yoi* and *yame* have no place in actual combat, but for the proper cultivation of the attributes sought after in the *do,* such things can be seen as essential.

Also, I think there may have been concerns that *kata* would be unnecessarily added to and embellished (when the exact opposite is really what is required).

Do not forget the employment or withdrawal of power, the extension or contraction of the body, the swift or leisurely application of technique (principle nineteen).

On the face of it, this seems to mirror principle fourteen, but we need to take it away from actual combat for a second and into the training. Is Funakoshi implying that by analysing the way speed (or lack of it) and body mechanics are employed on a technique we could find more than one use for it?

It would certainly make the committing of techniques to muscle memory easier if the biomechanics were the same for several interpretations. Looking again at my favourite kata of *Kanku Dai* and the profusion of *shuto* techniques within, this tends to make sense.

In simple terms, if you have a favourite strike, try and find a grappling alternative that employs the same physical movement, and vice versa, this will greatly reduce the chances of a "freeze" during an actual situation.

CONCLUSION: PART 1

Be constantly mindful, diligent, and resourceful in your pursuit of the way (principle twenty).

As a closer, Funakoshi gives us a catch-all comment reminding us to always bear the *do* in mind and to give it the attention it deserves. But he adds another word too: *resourceful*. This relates to an ability to quickly find ways to overcome difficulties and problems.

The problem practitioners of traditional karate face is that the *do* itself is coming second to people wanting pragmatic physical techniques. There isn't much of the *do* going on in your average MMA gym, and whilst their techniques are tried and tested, they are not (generally) balanced with the philosophy.

By showing the pragmatic side of traditional karate, it can be seen as still current and relevant and if, at the same time, we can begin to instil the values of the *do* into our students, this is not a departure from Shotokan, it is being resourceful as Funakoshi wanted.

Conclusion: Part 2

Your Karate-do

There are obvious parallels that can drawn between the formalisation of the Samurai arts following the Meiji Restoration, and what happened to karate when it was introduced to Japan. *Kenjutsu*, the art of the sword, for instance, became *Kendo* and *Iaido*, where the heritage was preserved within a formal setting and development of character became as important as learning the techniques. Over time, the ritual becomes the norm and the devastating effectiveness of the techniques becomes diluted, but all is not lost, and it only takes a few tweaks here and there to realise the full potential of the art.

So, what do we need to do to make our karate more pragmatic?

Make sure that the stances employed are used in the correct manner. You do not need a deep stance to apply power to a technique; you need proper body mechanics, the use of the hips and pushing the back foot into the floor will give you as much power (if not more) with your feet twelve inches apart as they would at full stretch, but you will be far faster across the floor and less of a stationary target. Deep stances are a fleeting physical response to an intentional lowering of gravity, for instance, during a throw. Get away from line training. Train by going back to *shizentai* after every technique or practising your techniques on the spot, similar to the way a boxer would.

CONCLUSION: PART 2

If the technique you are practising seems unnecessarily "flowery", strip it down. Think of what the technique seeks to achieve and take away any extraneous movement which does not assist you in accomplishing this. (Keep the applications realistic, however.)

If the "strike" seems unrealistic, or unnatural, look at it from a grappling point of view. In fact, try and find a grappling alternative for your favourite techniques. Karate is/was a holistic self defence system. Grappling, both vertically and on the floor, would have played a large part. Get out of your comfort zone, tinker and experiment.

Get away from the "formal" target areas of *jodan, chudan* and *gedan*. They are far too general. You need to be more specific in your targeting. Know what the best weapon for striking the chosen area is, and know the ramifications of delivering the blow. Learn human anatomy.

Learn the law regarding violence in the country where you live. Instructors need to realise and recognise the responsibility they take upon themselves when they teach serious combative techniques to others. Those learning the techniques need to realise the importance and possible ramifications of what they are being taught.

Take your training outside the dojo when it comes to concepts like *zanshin* and *mushin*. Cultivate mindful self-awareness. Follow the common sense principles included in this text to make yourself more aware.

Lose your ego. Bruised egos are responsible for the majority of violent encounters. Unless you need to get yourself out of a tight spot (which might have been avoided by adhering to the point above) ask yourself: Is it really worth it? Chances are that no, it is not.

You may notice, if you try the ideas in this text, that your karate may start to look like other styles. Your stances may look more like the fast shallow stances of Wado Ryu, or the grappling side might seem reminiscent of Goju Ryu. You may decide, after you have tried it, that it is not for you. You may even decide not to try it at all. Any of the above is ok, because we are all individuals. Even two practitioners of the same style with the same length of training under the same *sensei* will perform their karate in subtly different ways.

Physiologically, we are all the same, aren't we? Well, the short answer is no, we are not. Just as we are all born with different hair colour and skin tone, we are each the proud possessor of a unique physiological make up.

Scientists have tried to classify the human species (as scientists do) and come up with the endomorph, mesomorph and ectomorph, which are nothing more than guidelines for what "type" of person you might be when it comes to being fat, thin, or muscular and how easy it is for you to stay that way. But what makes you *you* is totally unique.

You may have injuries from when you were a child which affect the way you do things. You may have a congenital condition, such as asthma or a physical disability or some psychological condition. There may also just be something inside you that "clicks" with a certain way of doing things. You may find yourself more disposed towards grappling, or leaning towards striking and you will *definitely* find that you are better at some aspects of your karate than others, even if you are a good all-rounder.

So what are different styles of karate? They are merely the individual expressions of the founder based on the way they felt comfortable doing things. All the great masters were taught by someone else, who would have performed things slightly differently from the way their students eventually would. All *karateka* begin by learning a certain style, but eventually their karate becomes just that: *theirs*.

People who do not practise karate and have no real interest in it just see it as "karate". They do not see the different styles. Maybe we should also do the same. I cannot really say that the physical side of my training is pure Shotokan because I never trained under Master Funakoshi. The training I received was three or four steps removed from him. Even if I had received training from the man

CONCLUSION: PART 2

himself, we are physically poles apart. He was barely five feet tall, whereas I am six three. He was light, I am heavy. After he had taught me the basic techniques our physiological differences would mean that eventually I would find a way of executing them which suited my body type.

The one constant that can be carried from one generation to the next, regardless of physical differences or nuances in technique, is the philosophy. Funakoshi Sensei and others like him created a means whereby the training in karate can make us better people, with a philosophy of discipline, tolerance and restraint, and no impetuosity or violence. These characteristics seem to be sadly lacking in society these days.

So does it matter if you do not throw your kicks as I do? Does it matter if you borrow techniques, or even *kata* from other styles? No, it does not. Because the way you practise karate is yours, and yours alone.

One thing that should be consistent regardless of style or body type, is the *do*. There is an obsession these days with "street wise" techniques and, in this day and age, there is certainly a demand for it. People should have a right to defend themselves and be capable of doing so. The bulk of this text is about making training in traditional karate more streetwise. But effective training does not stop at the physical, there must be mental conditioning too.

So, in the end, what style you practise does not really matter. Whether your stances get shorter or your techniques get less "flowery" does not matter. As long as you carry the original philosophy and adhere to that in everything you do, you are not betraying your karate "heritage", merely interpreting it in your own way to fit it into your world.

Technically speaking, with the translation of the word *karate* as "empty hand", you could argue that any martial art, from anywhere in the world that does not use weapons can be construed as "karate".

CONCLUSION: PART 2

There are a number of fighting schools these days which have a variety of specialities. This is mainly due to the growth of MMA. They practice Muay Thai for their striking, jiu-jitsu for their ground game, wrestling for their takedowns, and anything else which they feel would give them an advantage in the Octagon.

There is no doubt that this breeds well-rounded fighters, but before you start looking outside your chosen art to fill any gaps you perceive in your "street effective" arsenal, take some time to revisit your own art. You may find the tools to plug the gaps right there, once you are looking at it the right way. Be prepared to tweak it to suit *your* needs, and *your* physique and mind set. Every person is unique. So it follows that their karate should be too.

Glossary

Although not an exhaustive list of martial arts terms, what follows is an explanation of the terminology used during the preceding text.

Age-uke – "rising block". Traditionally used to block *jodan* punches but is actually more effective as a forearm strike or clearing technique.

Aikido – a martial art developed by Morihei Ueshiba from the battlefield grappling art of *aiki-jutsu*. It is heavily influenced by his Buddhist beliefs and involves utilising the opponent's momentum against them in order to propel them away.

Ashi-barai – foot sweep. It is executed exactly as the name implies, the sole of the foot is driven into the ankle or heel of the opponent sweeping their feet from under them.

Bassai – *a brace of kata, Bassai sho* and *Bassai dai* from the Shotokan style. They are an intermediate kata, referred to as *Passai* in W*ado-ryu*.

Bunkai – along with *oyo* the study of the actual applications of *kata* techniques.

GLOSSARY

Bushido – the Code of the Samurai, similar to European Chivalry, it heavily influences the Japanese martial arts, many of which are derived from Samurai battle techniques.

Chudan – name given to the middle section of the body when referring to target areas.

Do – The "way". In martial arts terms it refers to the arts as an entire philosophical system rather than a mere physical endeavour.

Dojo- a term used for the training hall in the Japanese martial arts, literally a place for practicing the *do*.

Empei – the collective term for elbow strikes.

Fumakomi – a stamping strike, usually delivered to the prone body of a downed opponent.

Gedan – name given to the area of the body from the waist down.

Gedan-barai – a low level sweep of the arm, interpreted (most likely erroneously) as a hard block against a kick but more likely a percussive form of *tettsui* either aimed at the lower body of the opponent or at an opponent who has been brought down by a previous technique.

Gi – the uniform worn by a practitioner of the Japanese martial arts. At one time, they were all white or black, now all kinds of colours are acceptable.

Gichin Funakoshi – the "grandfather" of modern karate. Without him, it is highly likely we would never have had the chance to study it.

GLOSSARY

Gojushiho kata – a brace of *Shotokan kata*, *Gojushiho dai* and *Gojushiho sho* are understood to be amongst the most advanced, if not *the* most advanced Shotokan *kata*.

Goju-Ryu – Okinawan style of karate, "Goju" literally means "hard/soft" and combines hard linear techniques with more relaxed circular ones.

Gyaku-mawashi-geri – Hook kick. Thrown the opposite way to *mawashi geri*, the striking surface is normally the heel or the sole of the foot. In this text the idea is put forth that it actually a reaping technique meant to be employed against the legs.

Gyaku-zuki – a reverse punch usually thrown with the opposite arm of whichever leg is foremost.

Hangetsu – a *kata* from the Shotokan canon whose name means "half-moon". It comes from the stances and generally circular techniques which are use throughout the *kata*.

Hara - an area in the lower stomach, about three inches below the navel. Seen as the centre of balance in external terms and the storehouse for *chi* or *ki* (life force) in internal terms. Also known as *tanden* in Japanese and *tantien* in Chinese.

Heian Kata – the five *kata* produced by Itosu and derived from selected techniques from older *kata*. Called *Pinan* in *Wado-Ryu* they are usually the first kata taught to a new student, each one being progressively more difficult than its predecessor.

Hikite – the "pulling hand" which is usually seen placed upon the hip or across the torso of the *karateka* whilst their other arm is employed in a "block" or strike.

Hiraken – a "backfist" strike, usually employed as a snapping technique but can be employed as a sweeping backhand punch which penetrates deep into the target.

Hiza-geri – a strike with any part of the knee.

Iaido – a sword-based art which originated when *Kenjutsu* was formalised and employs very precise *kata* for the use of the sword which involve drawing it from the scabbard and cutting in a single movement. It is the ideal of the "one cut kill" and is a solo practice where precision of the various movements is seen as paramount. Usually undertaken in tandem with Kendo in order to preserve the combative aspect of *Kenjutsu*.

Ippon ken – a punch thrown with one knuckle protruding out further than the rest. Useful for striking soft tissue and extremely painful when used against the back of the hand or philthrum.

Ippon Kumite – "One step sparring" whereby a *karateka* will attack a fellow student with one attack. Once the other has defended themselves against the given technique, both return to *kamae* and the action is them repeated.

Jodan – name given to the region of the head when speaking of striking areas.

Judo – Literally "gentle way". Developed from jujitsu by Jigoro Kano, this employs the opponents strength as a tool against them to facilitate the use of throws and techniques for subduing them once on the ground. Now a phenomenally popular sport.

Judoka – a practitioner of *Judo*.

GLOSSARY

Jujitsu – the forerunner of Judo, this was a brutal system of fighting comprising both striking and grappling techniques, the nastiest of which were removed when Judo was invented. It was heavily adapted to become Brazilian jujitsu, a staple of MMA.

Jyu-kumite – Freestyle sparring with no formal stances and no named attacks.

Kamae – a ready stance. Usually involves moving into *shizentai* but some *kata* also have their own *kamae*. Similar to *"en garde"* in fencing.

Kanku-dai – A *kata* whose name means "gazing at the sky". Also eponymously named *Kushanku* after its founder. A favourite *kata* of the author.

Karate-do – the "way of the empty hand" which originated in Okinawa before being exported to Japan and thence the world. It employs a variety of strikes kicks and grappling techniques.

Karateka – one who practices karate.

Karate ni sente nashi – roughly translated this means "there is no first attack in karate". It is open to interpretation exactly what this entails.

Kata – Sometimes referred to as a "form", this is the Japanese name given to a set repertoire of certain techniques put together into a sequence and practiced in that order as a system for aiding retention and muscle memory.

Kendo – the formalised practice of sword based sparring, performed with *shinai,* or swords made from split bamboo. Usually undertaken in tandem with Iaido training.

Kenjutsu – the name given to the sword based fighting arts in Japan.

Keri – pronounced *"geri"*, it is the collective term for kicks in karate. The basic kicks all have a "snap" version or *keage* and a thrust version or *kekomi,* dependent upon the body mechanics employed and the purpose behind throwing the kick. The *keage* versions of *mae-geri* and *mawashi-geri* tend to be favoured over their *kekomi* counterparts in the West.

Kiba-dachi – the straddle or "horse" stance. This involves the *karateka* being sideways on to the opponent with legs about twice shoulder width apart and the weight distribution even between both legs.

Kihon – Quite literally "basics" and used in karate to refer to the practice of single techniques and their subsequent combinations.

Koan – a seemingly impossibly obtuse riddle employed in Zen Buddhism to promote deep thought during meditation.

Kokutsu- dachi – back stance. One foot pushed outwards to the front, the other turned ninety degrees to front and heels in line. The weight is relaxed over the back leg with a distribution ratio of approximately 60-40.

Kumite – the term used for sparring in traditional karate, whether formalised or "freestyle".

Kyokushin – a hard, competitive style of karate developed by Mas Oyama after he studied under a variety of martial artists, Funakoshi included. Oyama was an interesting man and a formidable *karateka.* A somewhat romanticised version of his life is the basis for the highly enjoyable film *Fighter in the Wind.*

GLOSSARY

Mae-geri – A kick thrown directly to the front, usually employing the ball of the foot as a striking surface but the instep and heel can be utilised also.

Makiwara – punching board, It is usually constructed from a plank of wood which has its thickness tapered and has the topmost portion wrapped in straw or similar padding. It is fixed into the ground and used to condition the striking surfaces of the *karateka's* body.

Mawashi-empei – a sweeping elbow strike which was somewhat neglected during traditional Shotokan practice when I was growing up but one which appears regularly in *kata* and one which every serious pragmatic *karateka* should be familiar with.

Mawashi-geri – round kick. A later addition to the arsenal of karate kicks but one which is hugely popular. The striking surface is either the ball of the foot or the instep and involves raising the knee and rotating the hips to assist in driving the foot into the target along a horizontal plane.

Mikazuki-geri – a crescent kick which involves raising the knee and then arcing the foot inwards across the body.

Mokuso – a period of meditation which takes place before and after karate training in order that the *karateka* can prepare themselves mentally for training, and then clear their minds at the conclusion of the training session.

Moroto-uke – traditionally executed as an "augmented block" and involves one arm sweeping across as in *uchi-ude-uke.* but the hand which would normally act as *hikite* is clenched into a fist and pushed into the side of the other arm's elbow. It appears quite a lot in *kata* and really seems to mimic pulling an opponent forwards and down before delivering a vertical *empei* to their exposed back.

GLOSSARY

M.M.A. – Acronym for Mixed Martial Arts, a collective term for techniques borrowed from several different styles and systems of fighting for use in sporting matches.

Muay Thai – also known as Thai Boxing, this is actually a highly effective Thai martial art with a long distinguished history and is far more than the sport many believe it to be. Its sporting aspect is generally regarded as the national sport of Thailand.

Mushin – literally "no mind" a state of complete mental clarity where the martial artist is fully immersed in the moment with no interfering thoughts or outside influences.

Naihanchi/Naifanchi – older *kata* from which *Tekki* originated (see *Tekki*).

Neikoashi–dachi – the stance from which *kokutsu-dachi* originated. Referred to as the "cat stance" it is basically a radically shortened version of the latter stance and is really a natural result of pulling away from an opponent whilst keeping the groin protected.

Nukite – a strike which employs the fingertips as a point of impact. It can be employed using all four fingertips, one finger *(ippon nukite)* or two fingers *(nihon nukite).*

Oyo – the term used, along with *Bunkai,* for the translation and interpretation of *kata* techniques.

Rei – quite literally "respect".

Sensei – Literally "one who has gone before". It is the term used to both address and describe an instructor in Japanese martial arts. It does not mean "master", as commonly thought.

GLOSSARY

Seppuku – ritual suicide adopted by the samurai used to atone for indiscretions and to regain honour through a noble death. It was also not uncommon for samurai leaders to commit *seppuku* if they were defeated and for vassals to commit *seppuku* in order to follow their feudal lord into the afterlife. It is sometimes crudely referred to as *hara-kiri*, which literally means "belly cutting".

Shizentai – the basic stance in karate where the practitioner stands with feet shoulder width apart. Used as a *kamae* before moving onto the other stances for *kihon* or *kata*.

Shodan – The Japanese term for first *dan* of first degree, the level attained when one first acquires the black belt. Subsequent *dans* continue in a similar vein *Nidan* (second), *Sandan* (third) etc.

Shotokan – a style of karate credited to Gichin Funakoshi. He also practised poetry and his pen name was "Shoto", "Shotokan", was the name for his dojo and hence his style.

Shuto – the edge of the hand as a striking surface.

Shuto-uke – often referred to as a knife hand block, it is actually a technique whereby a blow is delivered utilising the edge of the hand whilst the *hikite* pulls the opponent to the desired angle.

Sifu – the term used to address an instructor in the Chinese martial arts, the same way *sensei* is used for the Japanese.

Soto-ude-uke – a mid-level technique which was taught as a block but which is an extremely versatile movement which can be employed for a variety of combative scenarios. Opposite to *uchi-ude-uke, soto* sweeps from the outside inwards.

Sumo – an ancient form of wrestling from Japan which is highly ritualised and whose objective is to force your opponent out of a circle or cause them to place any other body part than the soles of their feet on the floor. Exponents reach gargantuan proportions but do not be fooled, despite their size and apparent obesity they are heavily muscled and extremely strong.

Sun Tzu – Chinese philosopher and strategist, author of *The Art of War*.

Tai Chi (full name *Tai Chi Chuan* or *Taijiquan*) – Although these days the majority of practitioners are interested in its benefits as a therapeutic exercise it is, when practised correctly, a devastatingly effective martial art.

Taiho-Jutsu – an art of arrest and restraint once employed by the *samurai* in relation to civilian prisoners. For a time this art was also employed by the police in England and Wales.

Tai Sabaki – an aspect of karate which concentrates on effective footwork and movement of the body in order to avoid techniques and place oneself in the prime position to deliver techniques of your own.

Tanden/Tantien – see *Hara*.

Teep – a front kick employed by practitioners of Muay Thai and MMA which is more of a push to keep the opponent at a certain range and off-balance rather than as a penetrative strike.

Tekki – the forename for a trilogy of *kata*, named *Tekki Shodan, Nidan* and *Sandan*. They were derived from a single *kata* named *Naihanchi* or *Naifanchi* and are unique in that the only stance they employ is *kibadachi* and techniques are executed back and forth along a straight line.

GLOSSARY

Tettsui – a hammer fist. Any strike in karate which employs the fleshy underside of the clenched fist as a striking surface.

Tsuki – the collective term for all hand strikes in karate.

Uchi-ude-uke – a mid-level technique which was taught as a block but which is an extremely versatile movement which can be employed for a variety of combative scenarios. Opposite to *soto-ude-uke*, *uchi* sweeps from the inside outwards.

Uke – the defender in pre-arranged sparring. It literally means "the receiver".

Ura-mikazuki-geri – a crescent kick which involves raising the knee and arcing the foot outwards away from the body.

Ushiro-geri – a thrusting kick sent directly backwards by the *karateka*. It is usually employed during line training after a spin but actually is faster, safer and far more effective thrown directly behind from a standing start.

Wado-Ryu – style of karate developed by *Hironori Ohtsuka*, who studied *karate* under Funakoshi but was also highly skilled in *Jujitsu*. He merged the two to form *Wado-ryu*.

Yamae – at the conclusion of a formal exercise the martial artist is given this command as an instruction to "stand at ease" but maintain *zanshin*.

Yoi – the instruction given by a *sensei* when he wishes the practitioner to prepare themselves to move into *kamae*.

Yoko-empei – an elbow strike performed out to the side along a horizontal plane.

Yoko-geri – side kick. Usually thrown from *kibadachi* by beginners but can be thrown from any stance by more advanced practitioners. The *kekomi* version is an extremely powerful kick.

Zanshin – a state of complete awareness, where the martial artist is alert to everything going on around them.

Zen – a sect of Buddhism where immersion in the present moment is pursued in depth through long periods of arduous seated meditation, known as *zazen*.

Zenkutsu-dachi – front stance. One leg is foremost and bent at the knee, the rear leg is almost straight. The weight is predominantly over the front foot with a rough ratio of 70-30.

Bibliography and suggested further reading

If I were to try and list every book I have read which has subject matter either directly or indirectly related to this text, I would have a bibliography ten times thicker than the text it appends and would be bound to miss something. I have been reading about martial arts since I started practising them over thirty years ago. I have therefore limited my list to either books to which I have directly referred in my own text or books which I believe are among the most instructional and inspirational.

A Book of Five Rings by Miyamoto Musashi, translated by William Scott Wilson. Published by Kodansha International (2002).
ISBN 978 – 4 – 7700 – 2801 – 3

Art of War, *The* by Sun-Tzu, translated by Ralph D. Sawyer. Published by Barnes and Noble Inc. (1994).
ISBN 1 – 56619 – 297 – 8 *casebound*
ISBN 1 – 56611 – 298 – 6 *gift edition*

Bubishi – The Bible of Karate translated with commentary by Patrick McCarthy. Published by Charles E Tuttle and Co. (1995)
ISBN 0 – 8048 – 2015 – 6

CHAPTER TWENTY ONE

Bunkai-Jutsu by Iain Abernathy. Published by NETH publishing in association with Summersdale Ltd. (2002).
ISBN 0 – 953 – 8932 – 1 - 9

Code of the Samurai by A. L. Sadler, a translation of **Budo Shoshinsu** by Daidoji Yuzan.
Published by Charles E Tuttle & Co (1988).
ISBN 0 – 8048 – 1535 – 6

Dead or Alive by Geoff Thompson. Published by Summersdale (1997). ISBN 1 – 873475 – 36 – 5

Gift of Fear, *The* by Gavin DeBecker. Published by Bloomsbury Publishing (1997). ISBN 978 – 0 – 7475 – 3835 - 6

Groundfighting Series, *The* by Geoff Thompson. Published by Summersdale (1996) as a six volume set:
Vol. 1 - Pins, The Bedrock   ISBN 1- 873475 – 82 – 9
Vol. 2 – The Escapes   ISBN 1 – 873475 – 71 – 3
Vol. 3 – Chokes and Strangles   ISBN 1 – 873475 – 76 – 4
Vol. 4 – Armbars and Joint Locks   ISBN 1 – 873475 –81 – 0
Vol. 5 – Fighting From Your Back   ISBN 1 – 873475 – 86 – 1
Vol. 6 – Fighting From Your Knees   ISBN 1 – 873475 – 91 - 3

Karate-do Kyohan by Gichin Funakoshi, Published by Kodansha International (1973). ISBN 0 – 87011 – 190 – 6

Karate-do My Way of Life by Gichin Funakoshi. Published by Kodansha International (1981). ISBN 0 – 87011 – 463 - 8

Karate-do Nyumon by Gichin Funakoshi. Published by Kodansha International (1988). ISBN 4 – 7700 – 1891 – 6

CHAPTER TWENTY ONE

Power of Now, *The* by Eckhardt Tolle. Published by Hodder & Stoughton Ltd (2005). ISBN 978 – 0 – 340 – 73350 – 9

Streetwise by Peter Consterdine. Published by Protection Publications in association with Summersdale (1997). ISBN 1 – 873475 – 52 – 7

Throws for Strikers: The forgotten throws of Karate, Boxing and Tae-Kwon-Do by Iain Abernathy. Published by NETH Publishing (2003). ISBN 10 – 0953893227.

Twenty Guiding Principles of Karate, *The* by Gichin Funakoshi translated by John Teramoto. Published by Kodansha International (2007). ISBN 4 – 7700 – 2796 – 6

Way of the Peaceful Warrior by Dan Millman, Published by H. J. Kramer/New World Library (2002) ISBN 0 – 91 – 5811 – 89- 8

White Ghost by Shaun Hutson, Published by Warner Books (1994) ISBN 0 – 7515 –0768 – 7

BV - #0144 - 230326 - C0 - 229/152/9 - PB - 9781909544574 - Matt Lamination